Treatment Planning for Traumatized Teeth

Treatment Planning for Traumatized Teeth

Mitsuhiro Tsukiboshi, DDS
Amagun, Aichi, Japan

quintessence books

Quintessence Publishing Co, Inc
Chicago, Berlin, London, Tokyo, Paris, Barcelona,
São Paulo, Moscow, Prague, and Warsaw

Library of Congress Cataloging-in-Publication Data

Tsukiboshi, Mitsuhiro 1952–
[Gaishoshi no shindan to chiryo. English]
Treatment planning for traumatized teeth / Mitsuhiro Tsukiboshi.
p. ; cm.
Includes bibliographical references and index.
ISBN 0-86715-374-1 (hard : alk. paper)
1. Teeth—Wounds and injuries—Treatment. 2. Periodontium—Wounds and injuries—Treatment: I. Title.
[DNLM: 1. Tooth Injuries—therapy—Atlases. 2. Tooth Crown—injuries—Atlases. 3. Tooth Injuries—diagnosis—Atlases. 4. Tooth Root—injuries—Atlases. WU 17 T8825g 2000a]
RK490.T7513 2000
617.6'0446—dc21

99-056647

Quintessence Publishing Co, Inc
551 Kimberly Drive
Carol Stream, Illinois 60188

First published in Japanese in 1998 by Quintessence Publishing Co, Ltd, Tokyo.

Printed in Japan.

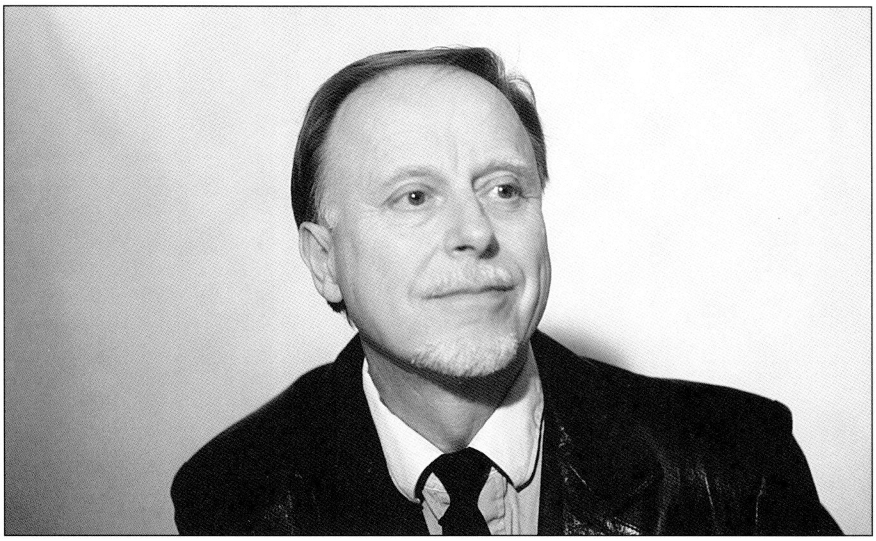

Dedicated to D. Jens O. Andreasen

I thank Dr Jens O. Andreasen, president of the International Association of Dental Traumatology and father of modern dental traumatology. I deeply respect him for his devotion to the study of improving the treatment of dental trauma. The success of the cases illustrated in this book could not have been achieved without his research and publications.

Special thanks to Dr Hirokazu Sanada, who helped with computer graphics, and Dr Leif K. Bakland for his assistance in editing the English edition.

Foreword

Significant improvements have taken place in all aspects of dentistry during the past quarter century. Improved treatment techniques, better materials, and heightened awareness of the benefits of prevention and the use of fluoride all have resulted in better dental health in many countries. Improvements have also occurred in the area of dental trauma: Increased knowledge of the outcome of treatment approaches, along with improvement in materials and techniques, has led to better management and more predictable results.

In this book, Dr Tsukiboshi emphasizes the importance of the three factors determining the prognosis of a traumatic injury: Accurate diagnosis of the extent and severity of the traumatic injury, the initial treatment of the acute aspect of the injury, and the long-term follow-up and treatment of sequelae to the injury. An important aspect often overlooked in other texts on dental trauma is the emphasis on avoiding unnecessary treatment procedures, particularly in the teeth of young patients. To this end, Dr Tsukiboshi describes clearly the biologic basis for healing after injury and the benefits of allowing normal healing processes to be used in the management of dental injuries. Overtreatment is to be avoided. With the current knowledge available in managing the traumatized tooth, the goal of this text is to provide guidance in saving teeth, restoring function, and improving esthetics after traumatic injury.

Leif K. Bakland, DDS
Associate Dean
Professor and Chair
Department of Endodontics
Loma Linda University
School of Dentistry

Contents

1

Anatomical Considerations

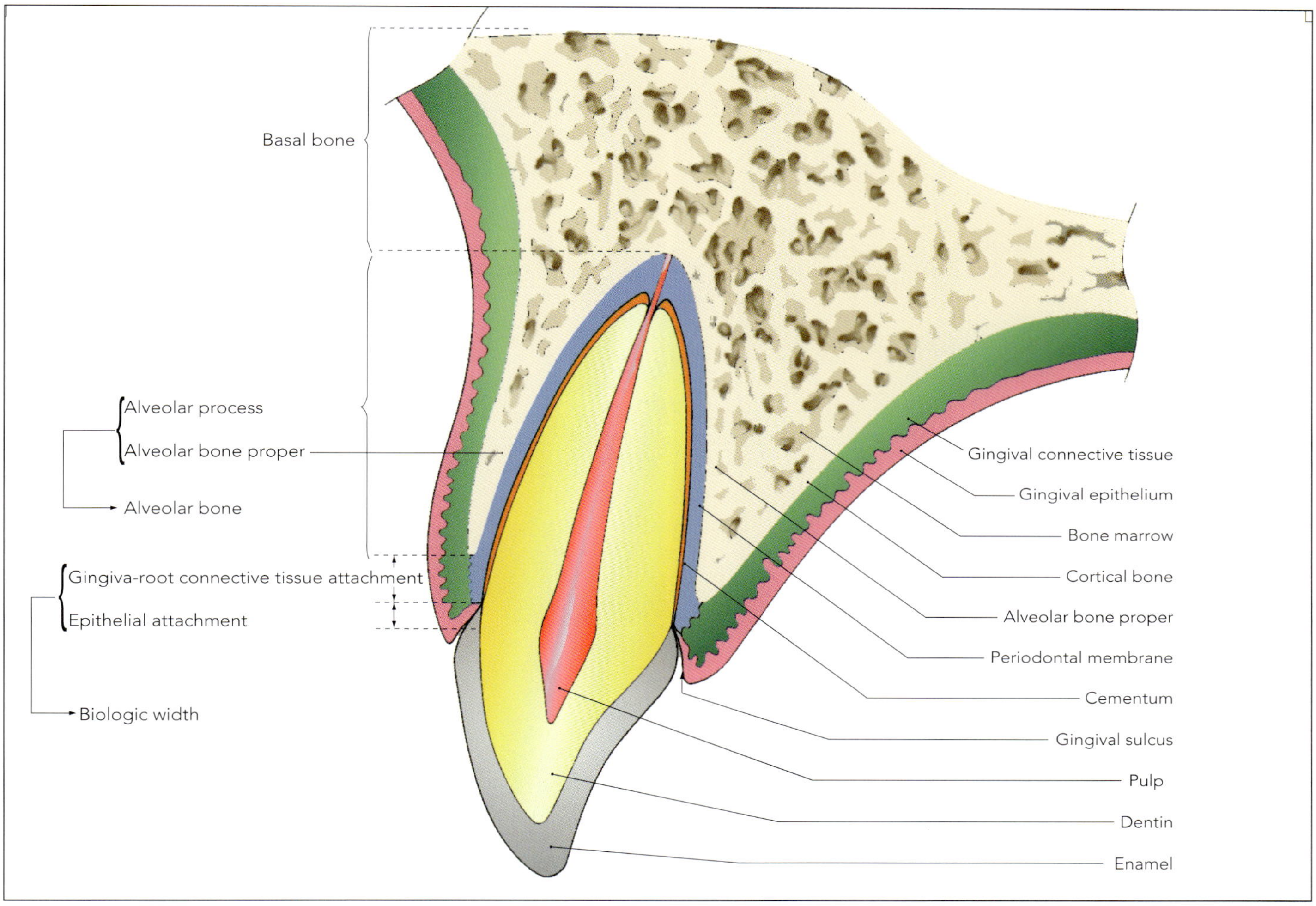

Fig 1-1 Tooth and periodontium.

Dentoalveolar trauma involves many tissues and structures. Recognizing the normal configuration of teeth and their supporting tissues is helpful when assessing the effects of trauma, planning corrective treatment, and evaluating the outcome.

A tooth consists of three hard tissues: enamel, dentin, and cementum. Dentin is formed by pulp cells, and cementum is formed by periodontal ligament cells (Fig 1-1).[1,2] Embryologically, the alveolar bone is composed of the alveolar bone proper and the alveolar process. The alveolar bone proper (linea alba, lamina dura) is the compact bone (cortical bone) within the alveolus and is formed by periodontal ligament cells.[3] The periodontal membrane lies between the alveolar bone and the cementum, and is connected to the tooth and alveolar bone or gingival connective tissue with Sharpey's fibers. This connective tissue attachment on the alveolar bone margin is usually about 1 mm wide, and the epithelial attachment is approximately 1 mm coronally. This 2-mm width is called the biologic width.[4]

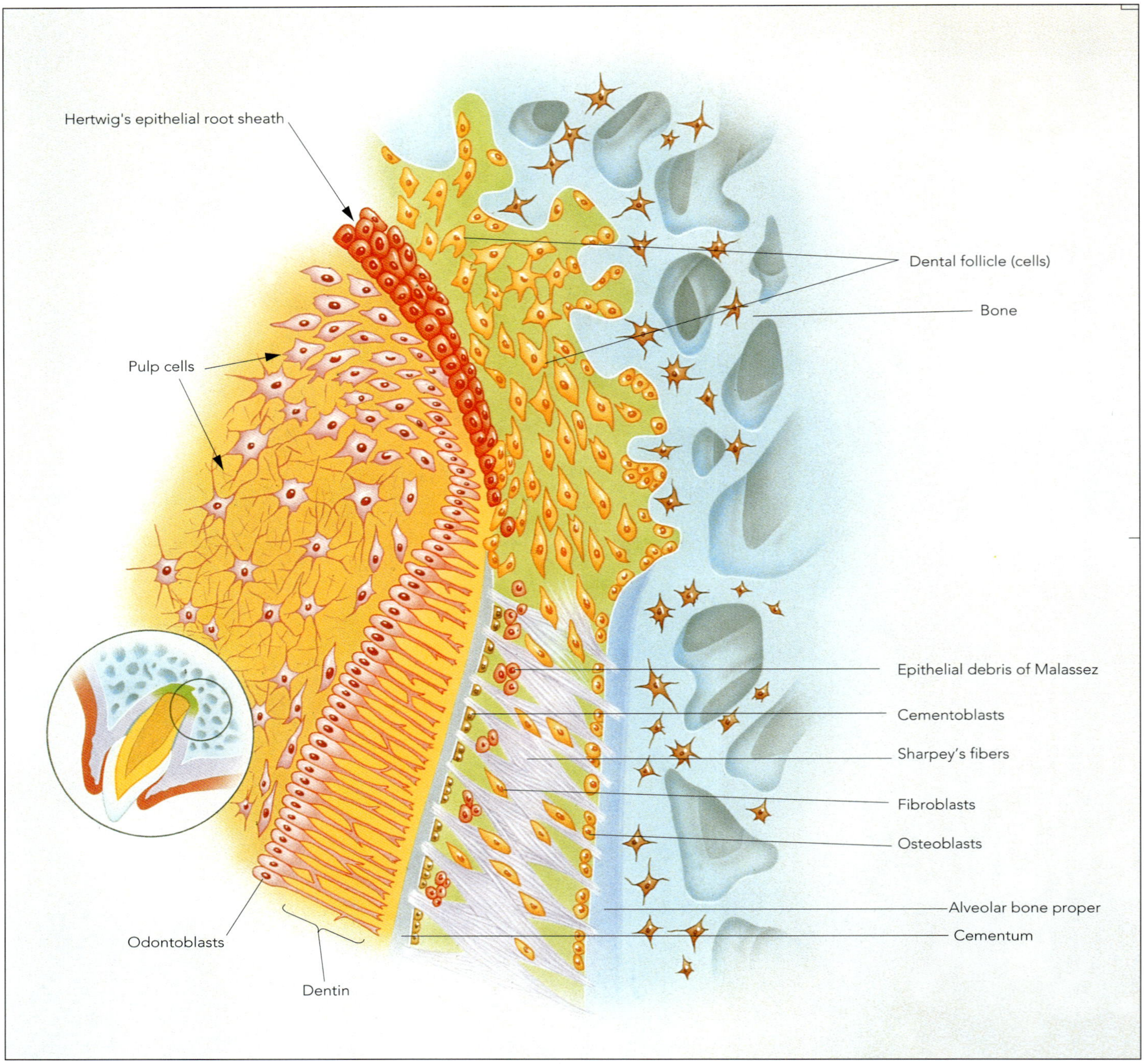

Fig 1-2 An immature root and periodontium around the apex.

A tooth with an immature root has Hertwig's epithelial root sheath in the apical region (Fig 1-2). Hertwig's epithelial sheath was originally the reduced enamel epithelium separated from the enamel. The reduced enamel epithelium is the tissue where inner and outer enamel epithelium combine. Hertwig's epithelial sheath plays an important role in root formation. On the pulpal side of the Hertwig's epithelial sheath, pulp cells are induced and differentiated to become odontoblasts; on the periodontal membrane side, cells of the dental follicle are induced and differentiated to become periodontal membrane cells (cementoblasts, fibroblasts, and osteoblasts).

2

Classification and Examination

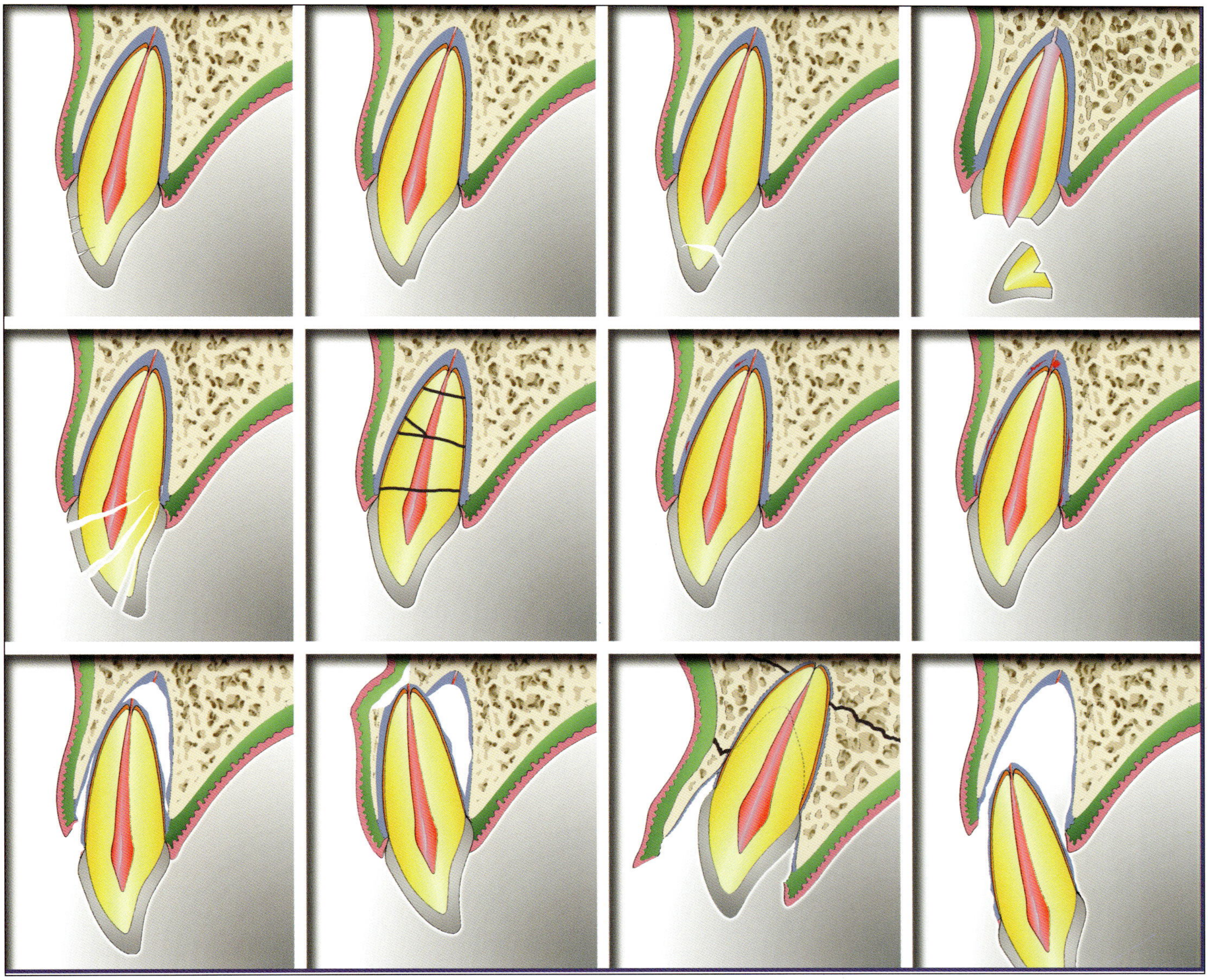

The classification of dental trauma used in this book is based on the World Health Organization (WHO) classification of diseases and has been modified according to Andreasen's recommendations.[5-7]

Fig 2-1 Classification

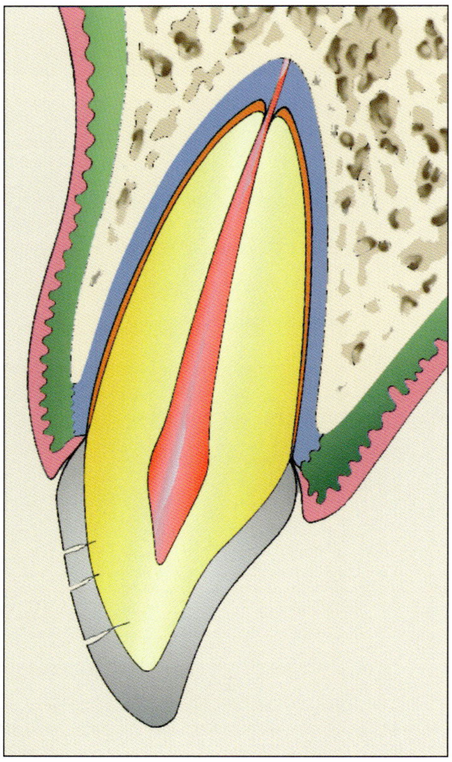

Fig 2-1a Enamel infraction.

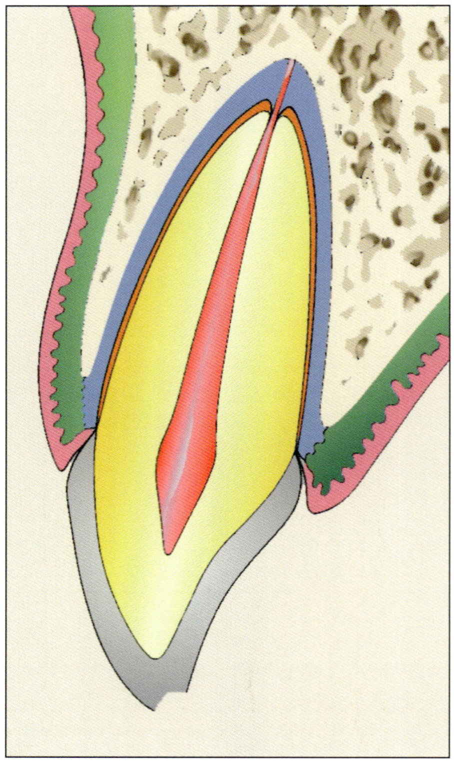

Fig 2-1b Enamel fracture.

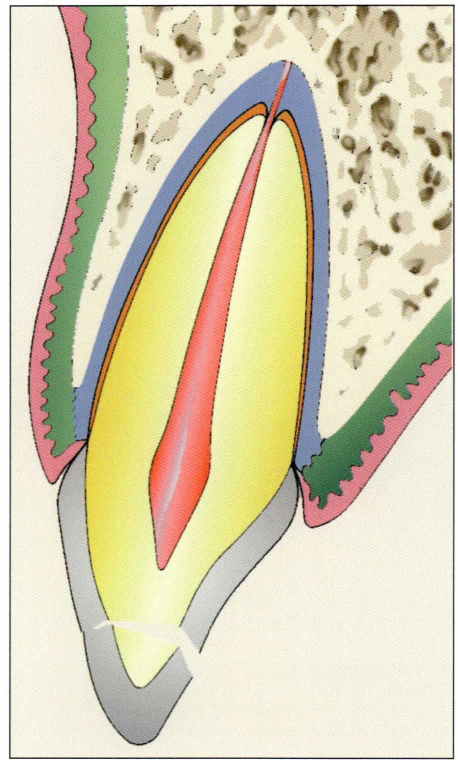

Fig 2-1c Crown fracture without pulpal involvement.

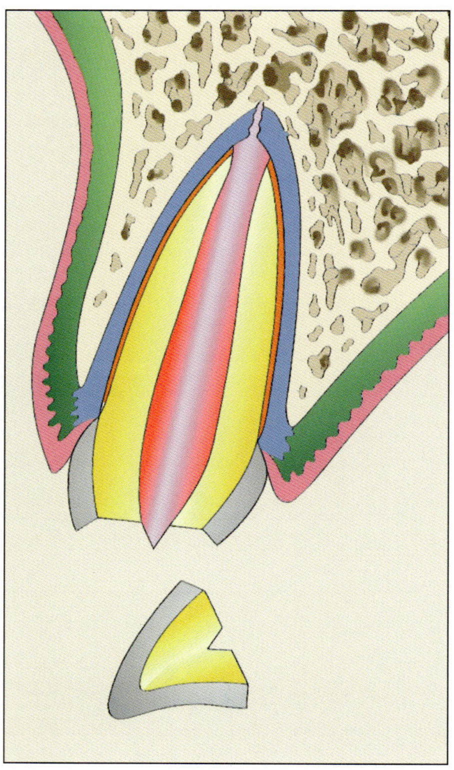

Fig 2-1d Crown fracture with pulpal involvement.

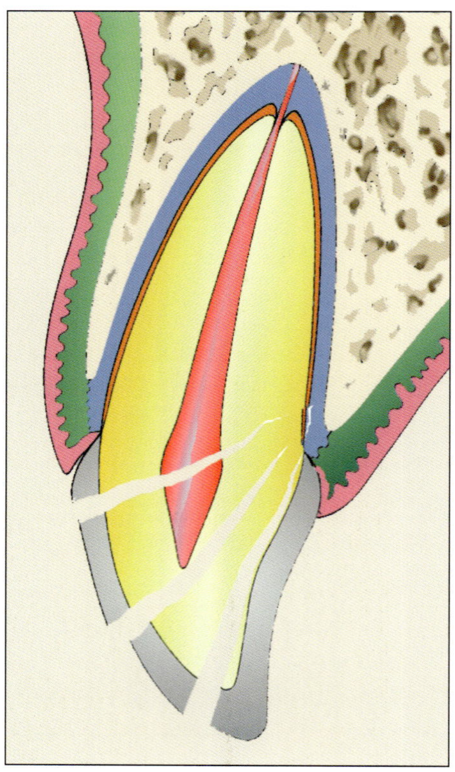

Fig 2-1e Crown-root fracture.

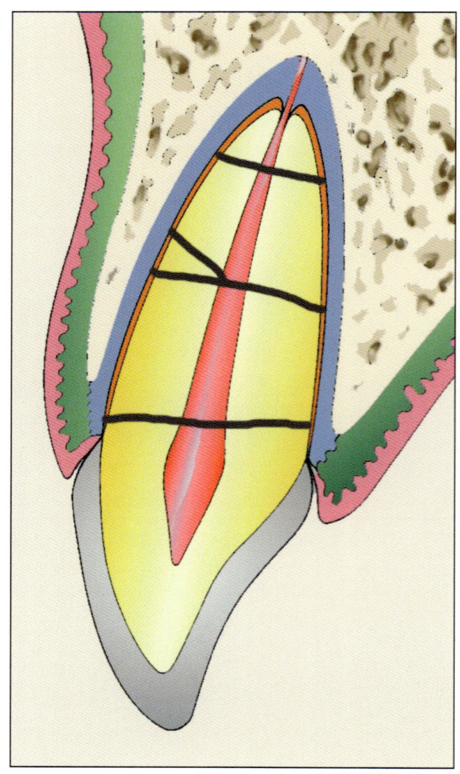

Fig 2-1f Root fracture.

Description

Traumatic force to the teeth or periodontium can cause destruction in a variety of directions and of a variety of magnitudes. Traumatic injuries are classified into various fracture and luxation types, but combination injuries often occur. For the sake of clarity, however, each type of injury will be described individually.

Enamel infraction and fracture

An incomplete fracture of the enamel without an enamel defect (crack) is called an infraction (Fig 2-1a). An enamel fracture is a small chip of enamel only (Fig 2-1b).

Crown fracture without pulpal involvement

This type of crown fracture involves only enamel and dentin with no direct pulp exposure (Fig 2-1c).

Crown fracture with pulpal involvement

This fracture involves enamel, dentin, and direct exposure of the pulp (Fig 2-1d).

Crown-root fracture

This fracture involves enamel, dentin, and cementum, and may or may not involve pulpal exposure (Fig 2-1e).

Root fracture

This fracture involves dentin, cementum, and pulp (Fig 2-1f). Special attention is required because root fracture and luxation injury may occur simultaneously (see Chapter 6).

Concussion

Concussion is a minor injury of the periodontium with no displacement of the tooth nor mobility (Fig 2-1g).

Subluxation

Subluxation is an injury of the peridontium without displacement of the tooth but with slight mobility. Damage to the blood supply of the pulp and the periodontium is usually minor, but pulpal problems occasionally result (Fig 2-1h).

Extrusive luxation

This injury is displacement of the tooth in an extrusive direction involving the periodontal support and the pulpal blood supply (Fig 2-1i).

Lateral luxation

The tooth is displaced from its long axis, usually with the apical end displaced labially and the coronal part palatally. The pulpal blood supply is usually completely severed (Fig 2-1j).

Intrusive luxation

This most serious of luxation injuries results in the tooth being displaced apically, leading to a crushing of the neurovascular bundle entering the pulp and severe damage to the cementum and periodontium (Fig 2-1k).

Avulsion

An avulsed tooth is completely displaced from the alveolus with total disruption of the pulpal blood supply (Fig 2-1l).

Fig 2-1 Classification (continued)

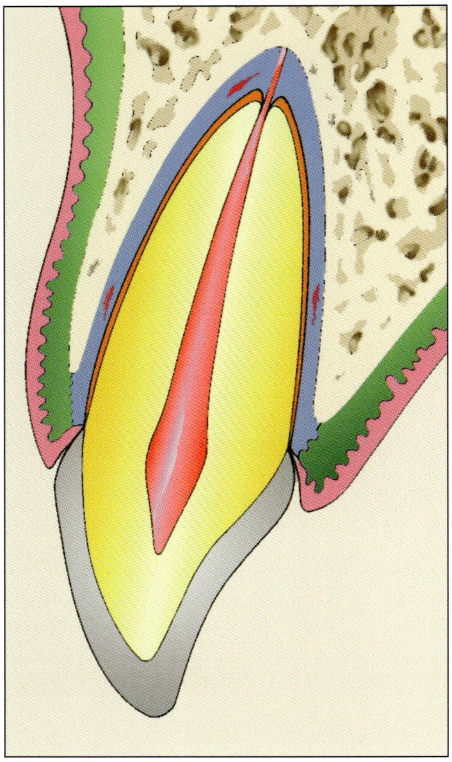

Fig 2-1g Concussion.

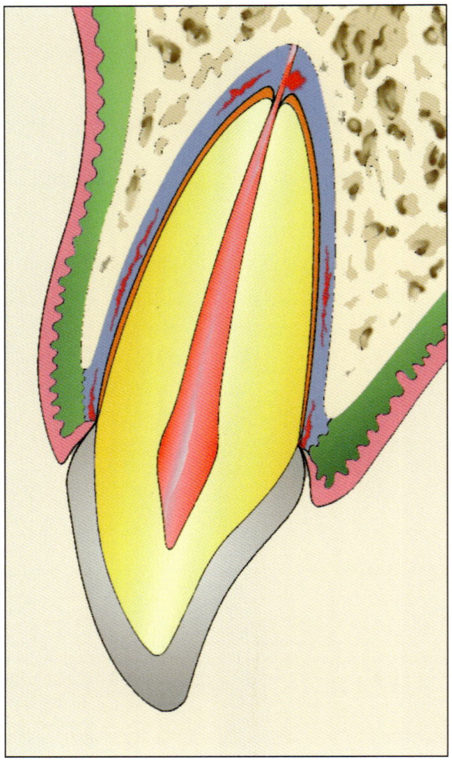

Fig 2-1h Subluxation.

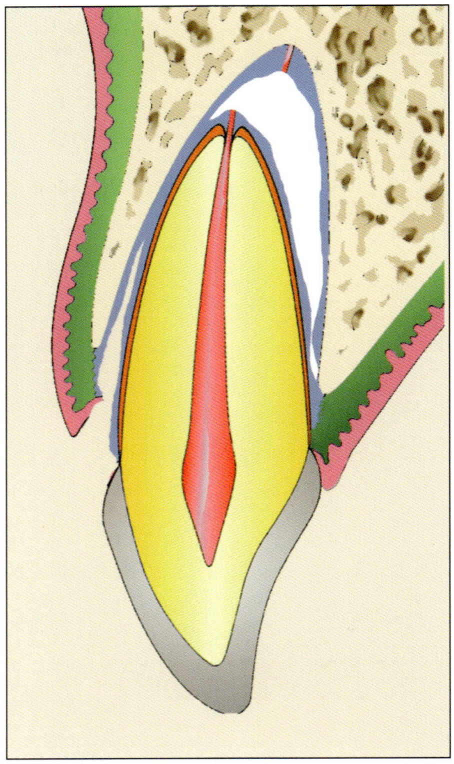

Fig 2-1i Extrusive luxation.

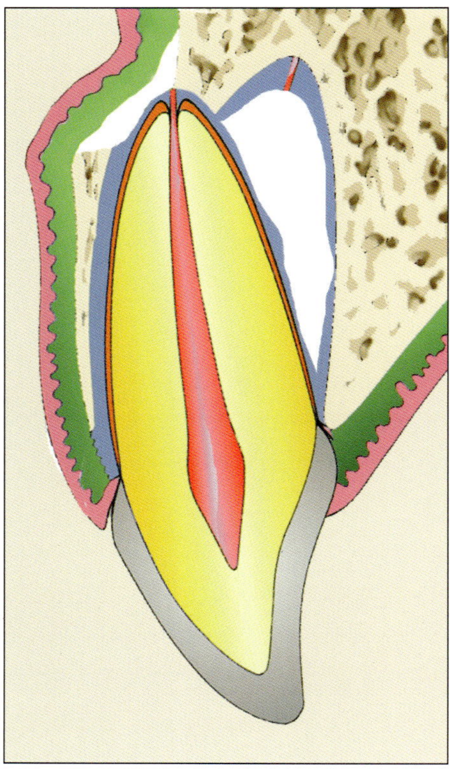

Fig 2-1j Lateral luxation.

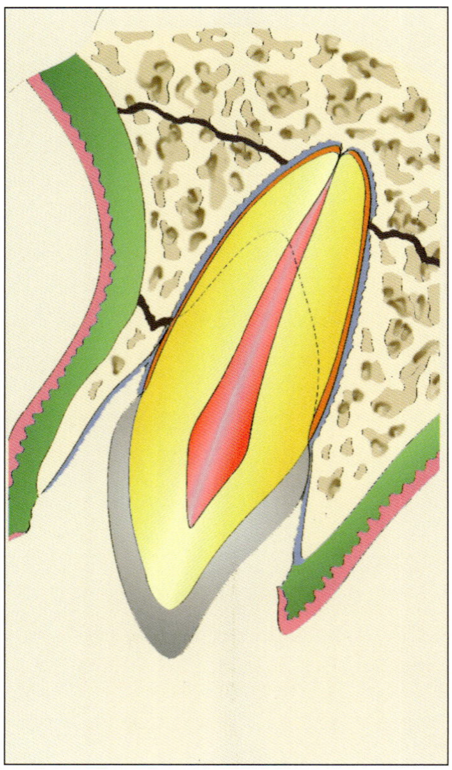

Fig 2-1k Intrusive luxation.

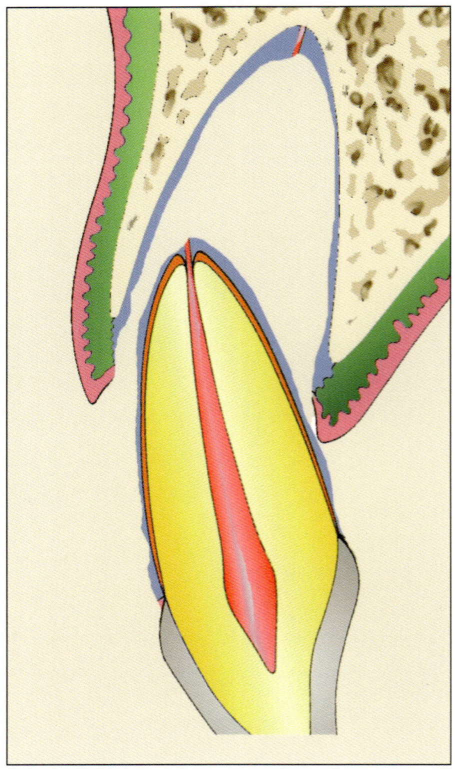

Fig 2-1l Avulsion.

Soft tissue injury and fracture of alveolar bone

Soft tissue injury involves the gingiva, oral mucosa, and lips. Fractures involve the alveoli and the jaw bones.

Examination and Diagnosis: Key Points

The patient's history and the findings of the clinical and radiographic examinations are the basis for proper evaluation of a traumatic injury. It is important to perform these examinations quickly and properly and to understand the nature of the injuries to teeth, periodontal membrane, and pulp.

Figure 2-2 is a sample record for traumatized teeth. This record facilitates complete examination and the development of a correct diagnosis and appropriate treatment plan. It also serves as a valuable reference at follow-up evaluations.

Patient history

Obtain pertinent information such as when, where, and how the injury occurred from the patient or attendant. When treating traumatized teeth, it is important to record the time of the accident and treatment date because this information may affect the prognosis. Identify the part of the oral cavity involved and the extent of dental injury. If the patient or attendant calls to report an injury, ask that any tooth fragment or avulsed tooth be brought to the office. Milk is a good storage medium for an avulsed tooth. If there is a possible loss of consciousness, a neurologic examination should be done before dental treatment. A carefully recorded history of trauma will help differentiate between symptoms and clinical findings from the present injury versus any previous injuries.

Is the patient able to chew? If not, there could be a bony fracture, which is often associated with malocclusion, even with no malposition of individual teeth.

Clinical examination

Intraoral examination includes inspection, palpation, thermal testing, and the electric pulp test (EPT). First, inspect any laceration of soft tissue and the degree of bleeding (Figs 2-3, 2-4, and 2-7). If there is bleeding or contamination, cleanse the injured area and re-examine the tissues. Next, confirm and record tooth fractures, malposition, missing teeth, and the presence of pulp exposure (Figs 2-3, 2-4, and 2-7). Recording the presence of tooth discoloration is an important procedure for postoperative observation (Fig 2-5). During palpation, check for mobility and percussion pain; also take note of any spontaneous pain. Mobility is an indicator of the degree of luxation.

Check pulpal response (ice and EPT). The EPT is important whenever pulpal trauma is suspected in order to detect teeth with pulp necrosis (Fig 2-5).

Record the various clinical findings and take intraoral photographs for complete records.

Radiographic examination

A radiographic examination is essential to detect and confirm fracture and malposition of teeth and bony fractures. Radiographs are needed for diagnosis of root fractures (Fig 2-4b and Figs 2-6c and d), recognition of subluxation and extrusive luxation (Figs 2-5b and 2-7b), and confirmation of tooth intrusion (Fig 2-7c) and alveolar bone fracture (Fig 2-7b). Sometimes it is necessary to take radiographs from different angles for an accurate examination, depending on the kind of malposition (eg, lateral luxation) and fracture (eg, root fracture) of the teeth. Root fracture can be confirmed by radiographs after a few months (Fig 2-6d). Also, inspect for embedded fragments of teeth and foreign bodies in soft tissues (Figs 2-4c and d). The treatment plan for the pulps of traumatized

Record of Traumatized Teeth

Patient's name: ______________________ Date of birth: ______________
❑ Male ❑ Female Age: ______________

Initial examination date: ______________ Referring dentist (or physician): ______________

Past trauma, if any
Date: ______________ Teeth involved: ______________

Present trauma
Date: ______________ Place: ______________
Cause: ____
____

General findings
Headache: ❑ Yes ❑ No Consciousness: ❑ Clear ❑ Not clear Nausea: ❑ Yes ❑ No

Intraoral findings
Teeth involved: ❑ Primary ______________ ❑ Permanent ______________
Spontaneous pain: ❑ Yes ❑ No Pain to ice: ❑ Yes ❑ No
Percussion pain: ❑ Yes ❑ No Pulp exposure: ❑ Yes ❑ No
Electric pulp test (EPT): ________
Discoloration of crown: ❑ Yes ❑ No Teeth mobility: ❑ None ❑ +1 ❑ +2 ❑ +3
Damage: ❑ to oral mucosa ❑ laceration of the lips ❑ other______________

Radiographic findings
Completion of root formation: ❑ complete ❑ incomplete (apical foramen ________mm)
Root fracture: ❑ Yes ❑ No Apical lesion: ❑ Yes ❑ No
Obliteration of pulp cavity: ❑ Yes ❑ No Root resorption: ❑ Yes ❑ No
Type of root resorption: ❑ surface ❑ inflammatory ❑ replacement
Widening of periodontal membrane (luxation): ❑ Yes ❑ No
Fracture of alveolar bone: ❑ Yes ❑ No

Condition of avulsed tooth
Duration of time out of oral cavity: (________minutes)
Stored in: ❑ dry ❑ in tap water ❑ in saliva ❑ in milk

Diagnosis
❑ crown fracture ❑ crown-root fracture ❑ root fracture
❑ concussion ❑ subluxation ❑ extrusive luxation
❑ intrusive luxation ❑ avulsion

Treatment plan

Prognosis

Fig 2-2 Sample record of traumatized teeth.

Fig 2-3 Case 1

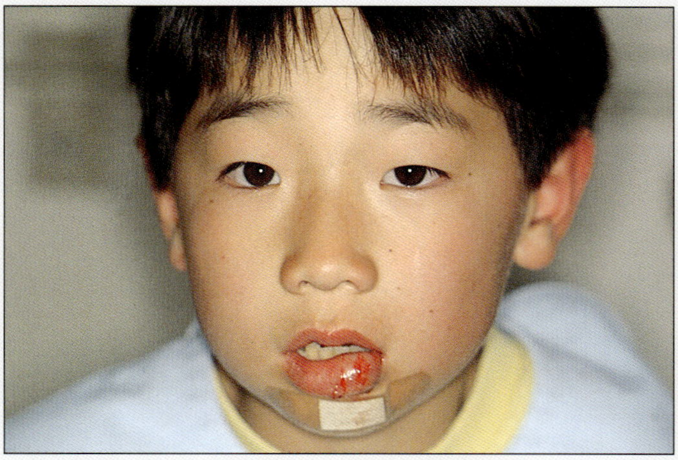

Fig 2-3a A 9-year-old boy fell and hit his anterior teeth during a ball game.

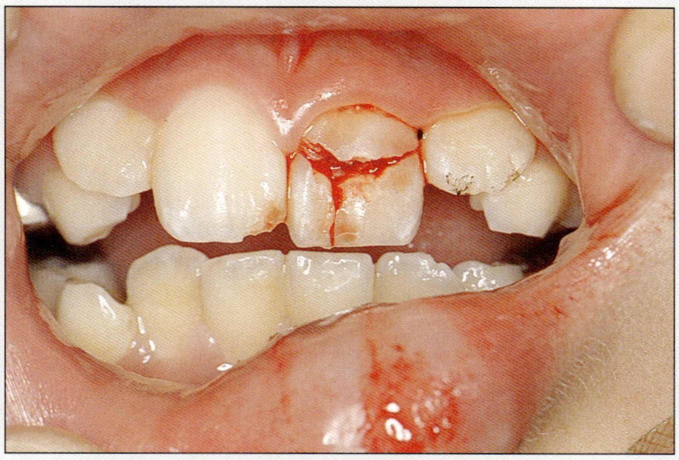

Fig 2-3b Note the contusion of the lower lip and crown fracture of tooth 9. Because the fractured fragments are still attached, there is a possibility of a crown-root fracture.

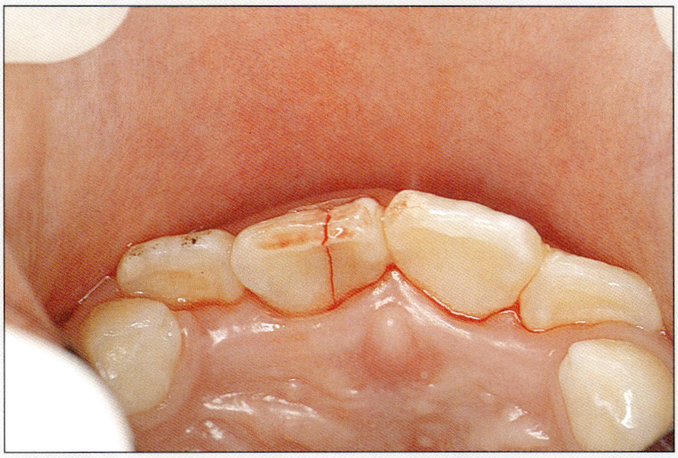

Fig 2-3c The fracture line reaches subgingivally on the palatal aspect.

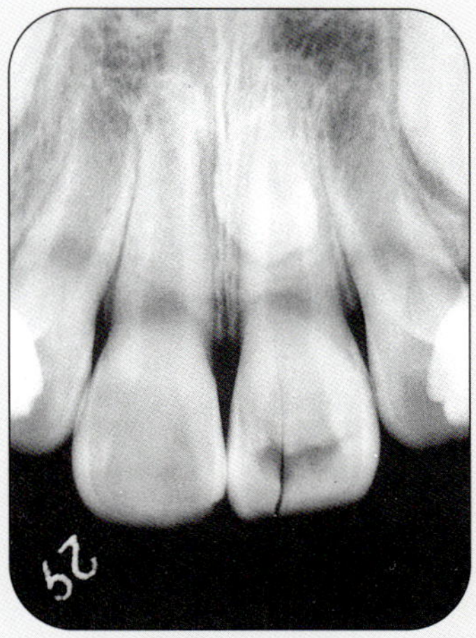

Fig 2-3d The fracture line extends below the crestal bone margin. The diagnosis is crown-root fracture.

teeth is affected by the degree of completion of the root formation, so this should be determined by radiographic examination. During postoperative observation, obliteration of the pulp cavity and the existence of root resorption should be carefully monitored.

Because radiographic examination is such an important part of the examination and diagnosis of traumatized teeth, it is important to take high-quality radiographs.

Other factors in examination

In the case of avulsed teeth, it is important to determine the length of time that the teeth have been out of the mouth and, if stored, the medium used. Milk is better than water for preserving the vitality of the cells on the root surface, an important factor in the successful outcome of replantation.

Only after thorough examination can the diagnosis and a proper treatment plan be made.

Fig 2-4 Case 2

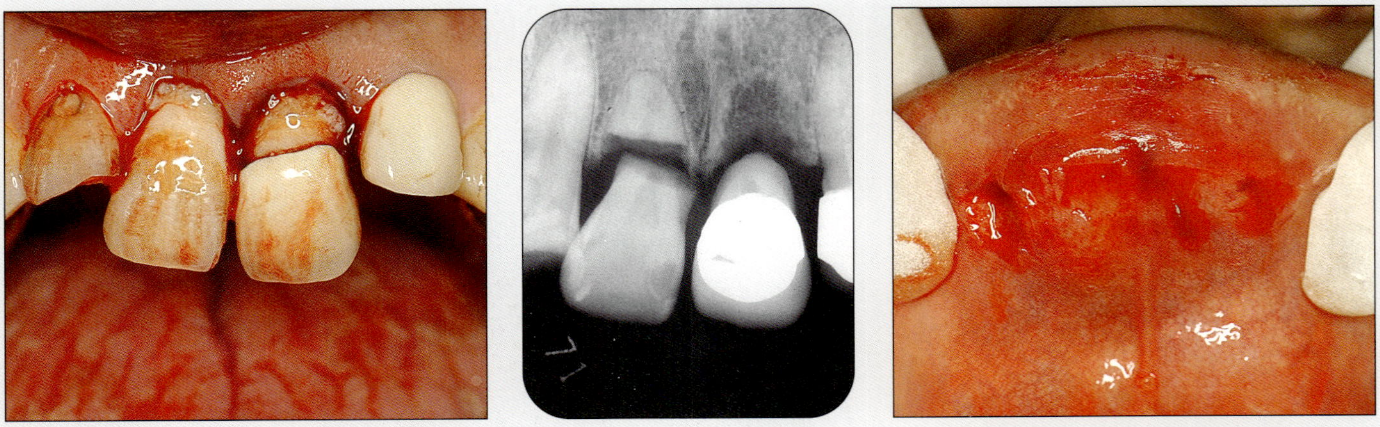

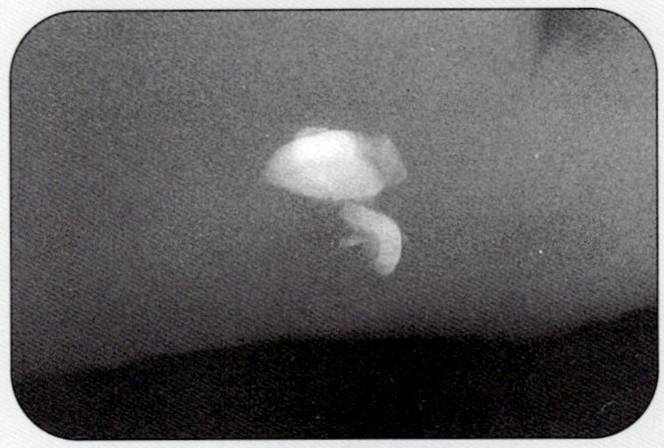

Fig 2-4a A 38-year-old man hit his lower face with a tool while gardening. He did not lose consciousness.

Fig 2-4b Intraoral examination and radiographs reveal crown fracture, root fracture, and extrusion. A previous trauma was suspected from the shape of the root (tooth 9) and the condition of the pulp cavity.

Fig 2-4c Palpation of the lips indicates an embedded foreign body in the lacerated area of the upper lip.

Fig 2-4d Radiograph of the upper lip reveals the presence of the fractured chip from tooth 7.

Fig 2-5 Case 3

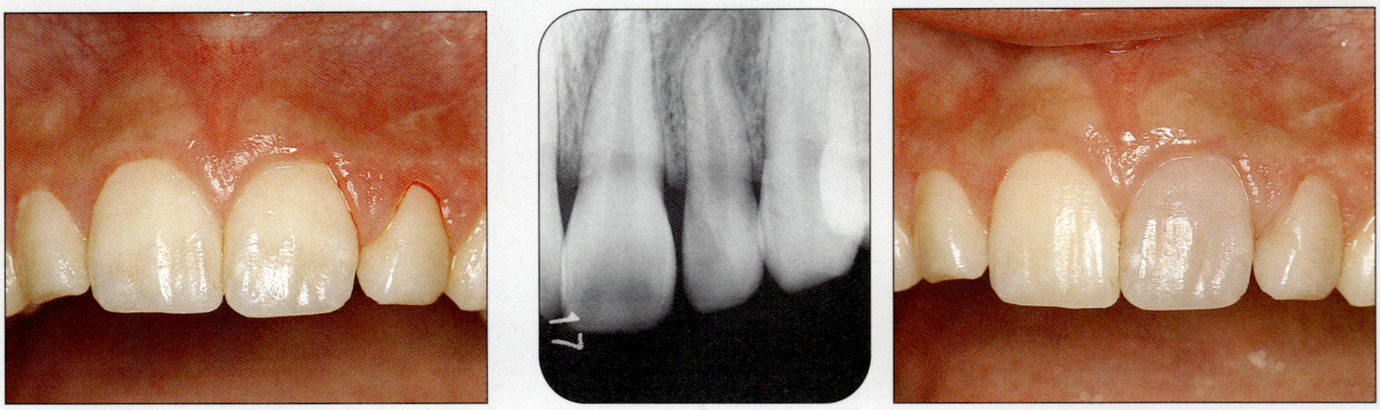

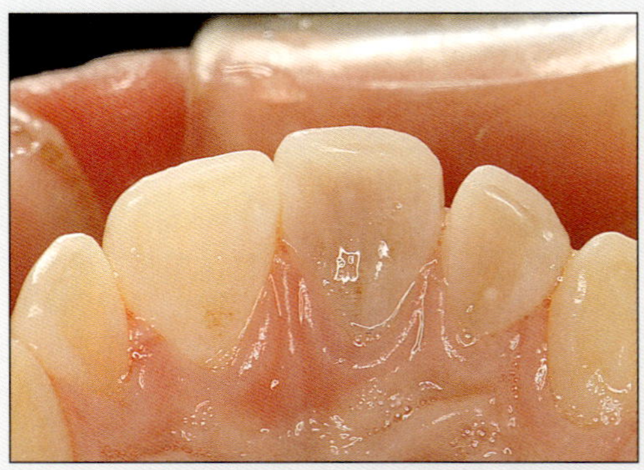

Fig 2-5a A 14-year-old boy fell and hit teeth 9 and 10. Inspection and palpation reveal slight bleeding from the gingival sulcus of teeth 9 and 10 and slight mobility. There was no response to the EPT.

Fig 2-5b The radiograph reveals no obvious widening of the periodontal membrane space.

Figs 2-5c and d One month later, there is noticeable discoloration of tooth 9 and slight discoloration of tooth 10. Diagnosis: subluxation resulting in disruption of the blood supply to the pulps.

Fig 2-6 Case 4

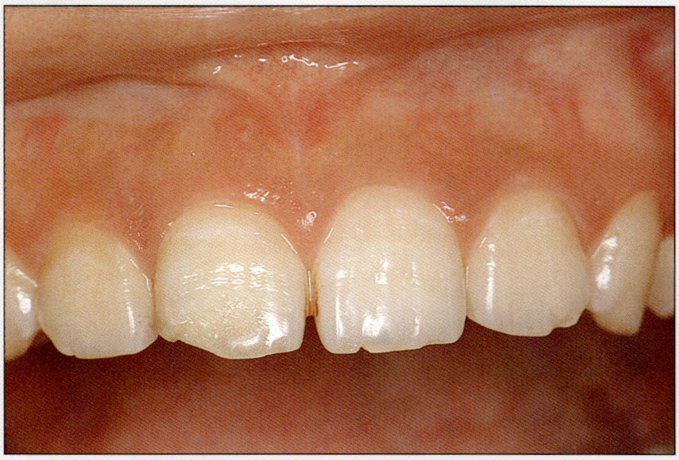

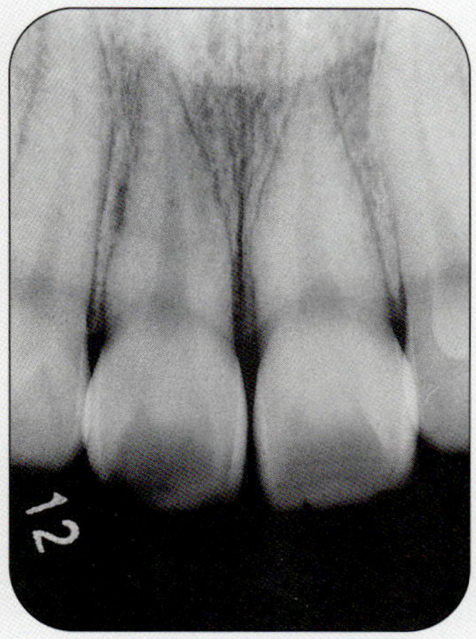

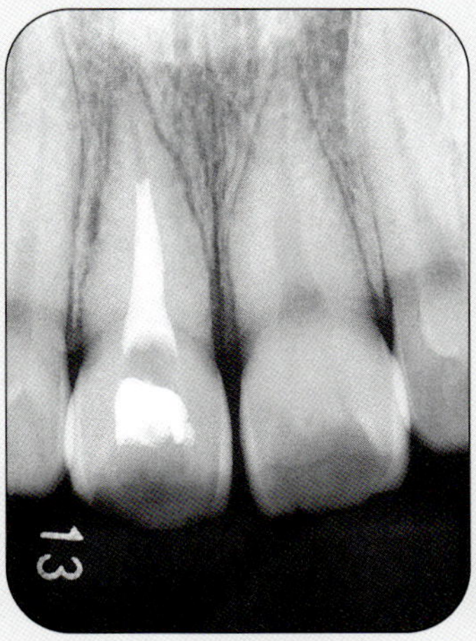

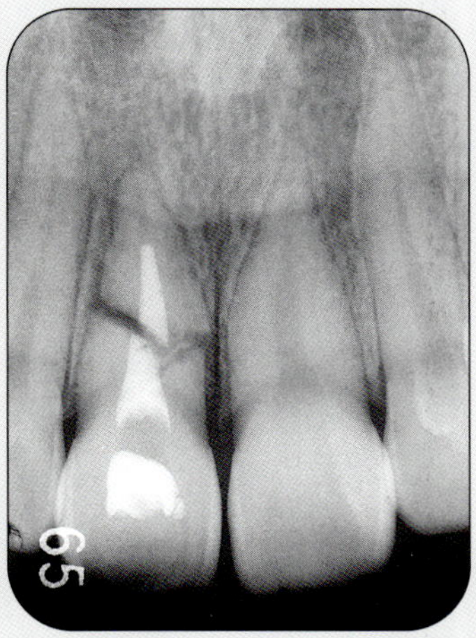

Figs 2-6a and b An 18-year-old woman sustained a mandibular injury in an automobile accident. There was a small crown fracture of tooth 8. Two months later, a slight discoloration of the crown and pain on percussion were observed. Pulp necrosis due to subluxation of tooth 8 was suspected.

Fig 2-6c The necrotic pulp was extirpated and the canal filled with calcium hydroxide.

Fig 2-6d Five months after the initial examination, a radiograph reveals a root fracture.

Fig 2-7 Case 5

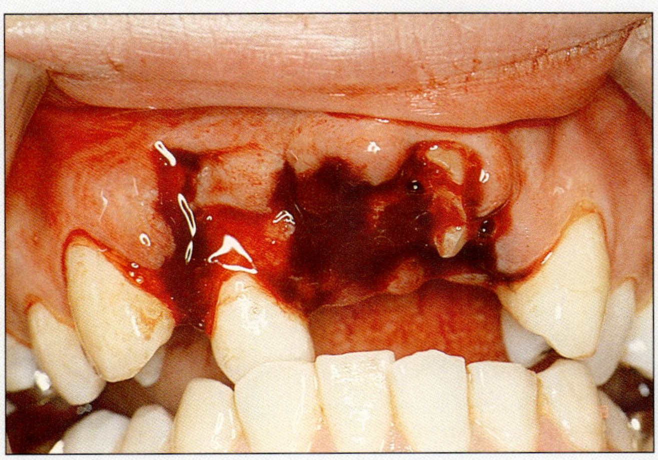

Fig 2-7a A 32-year-old woman sustained a severe facial injury in an automobile accident. Three hours elapsed before she sought treatment.

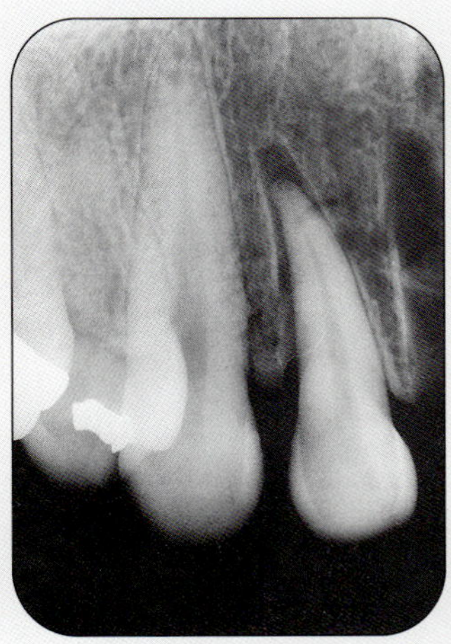

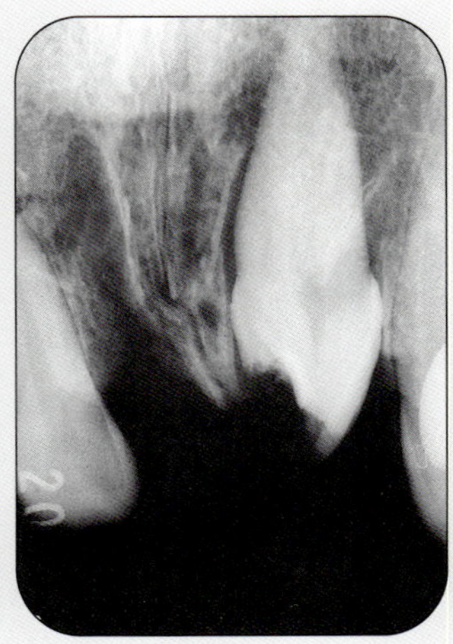

Figs 2-7b and c The radiographs reveal extrusive luxation of tooth 7, fracture of the alveolar bone, avulsion of teeth 8 and 10, and intrusive luxation of tooth 9.

3

Crown Fracture

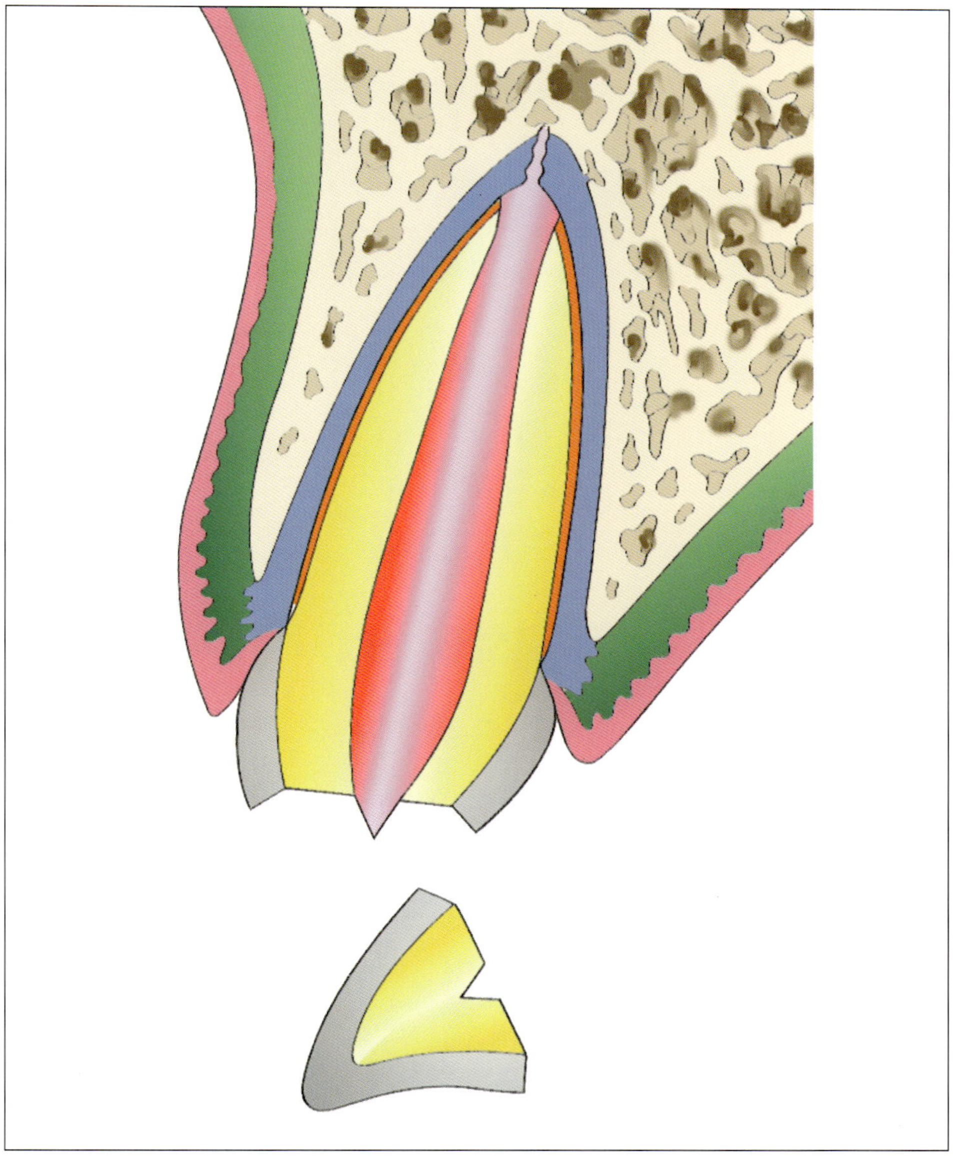

Crown fractures may involve enamel only, enamel and dentin, or enamel, dentin, and pulp. It should be remembered that any type of crown fracture may also be combined with a luxation injury.

Fig 3-1 Types of crown fractures

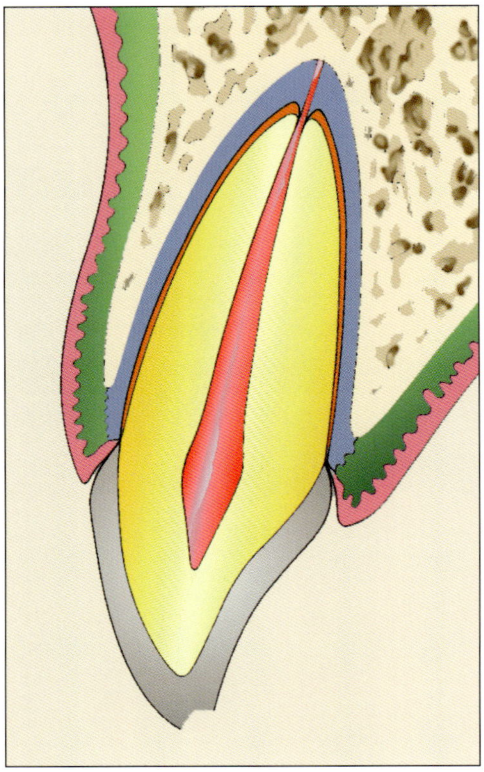

Fig 3-1a Enamel fracture.

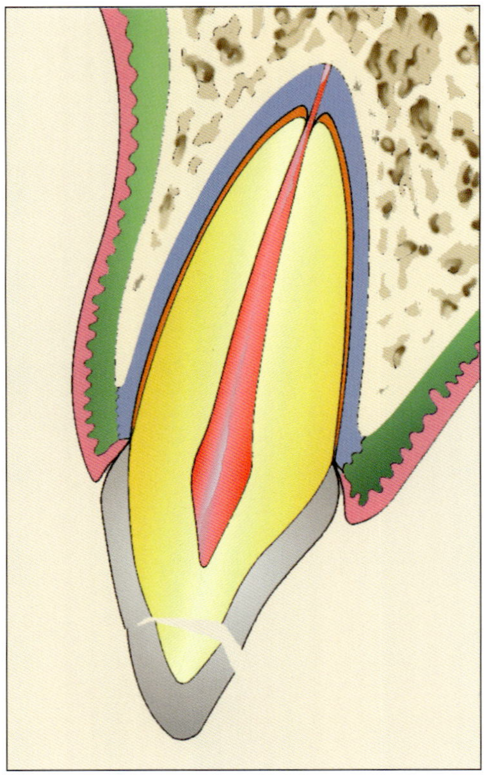

Fig 3-1b Uncomplicated crown fracture, involving enamel and dentin.

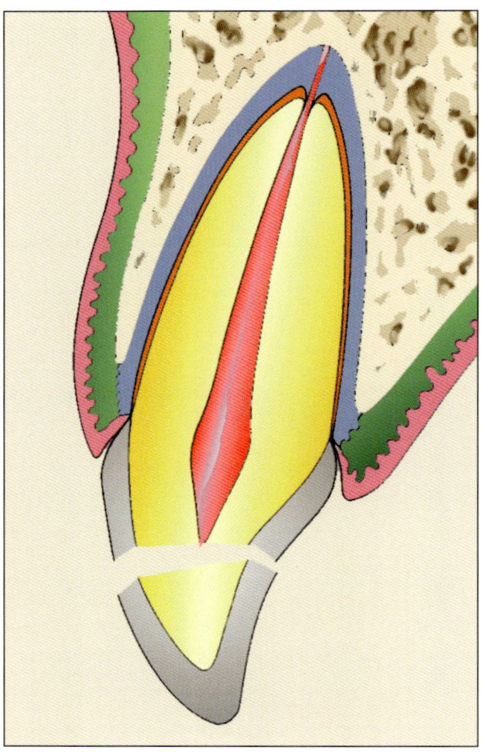

Fig 3-1c Complicated crown fracture, involving enamel and dentin and exposing the pulp.

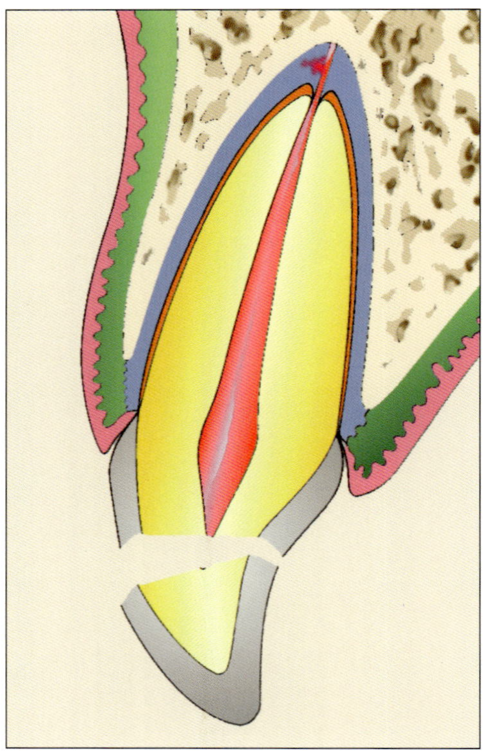

Fig 3-1d Crown fracture combined with luxation.

Description

Enamel fracture

An enamel fracture is limited to the enamel and includes enamel chips and infractions (Fig 3-1a).

Uncomplicated crown fracture

This fracture is limited to the enamel and dentin without pulp exposure (Fig 3-1b).

Complicated crown fracture

This fracture involves enamel and dentin with pulp exposure (Fig 3-1c).

Crown fracture combined with luxation

Ischemic changes in the pulp or pulp necrosis can occur as a result of concomitant luxation injuries (Fig 3-1d).

Examination and Diagnosis: Key Points

It is important to determine the extent of the fracture, whether the fracture is limited to the enamel and dentin, availability of the fractured fragment, whether the pulp is exposed, and if there is necrosis of the pulp. Palpate for soft tissue or bony injuries, and perform a radiographic examination and an electric pulp test (EPT).

Treatment Plan

Enamel fracture

For a small fracture, polish or selectively grind the fracture (Fig 3-2). For more extensive defects, restore with composite resin.

Uncomplicated crown fracture

If the tooth fragment is not available, restore the tooth with composite resin (Fig 3-3). If the tooth fragment has been saved, attempt to reattach it[8] (Fig 3-4). If the fragment is close to the pulp, consider pulp protection with a calcium hydroxide liner.

Complicated crown fracture

If the pulp exposure is very small, clean the exposed area and apply pulp capping to the exposed pulp (Fig 3-5). For a larger pulp exposure, partial pulpotomy should be performed. After cleansing and hemostasis, apply pulp dressing (Fig 3-6). The restoration should be done in accordance with standard procedure. If a material such as calcium hydroxide preparation or a composite resin is used for pulp capping, restorative treatment and pulp capping can be performed on the same day.

Crown fracture combined with luxation

Foremost, restorative treatment should be performed in accordance with current standard procedures. If after a few months there is no vital response from the pulp, perform root canal treatment. In most cases of pulp necrosis following traumatic injuries to young patients, apexification is the first choice (Fig 3-7). But for adult teeth with completely formed roots, endodontic treatment should be done, followed by restorative treatment.

Fig 3-2 Treatment of enamel fracture

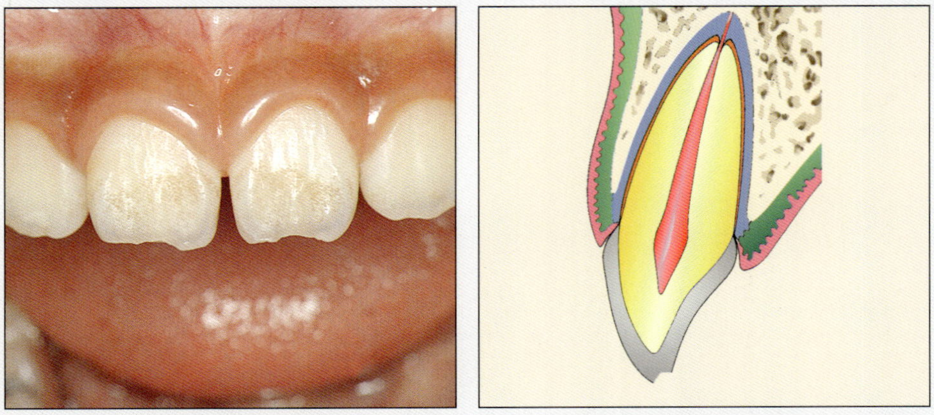

Figs 3-2a and b Preoperative view.

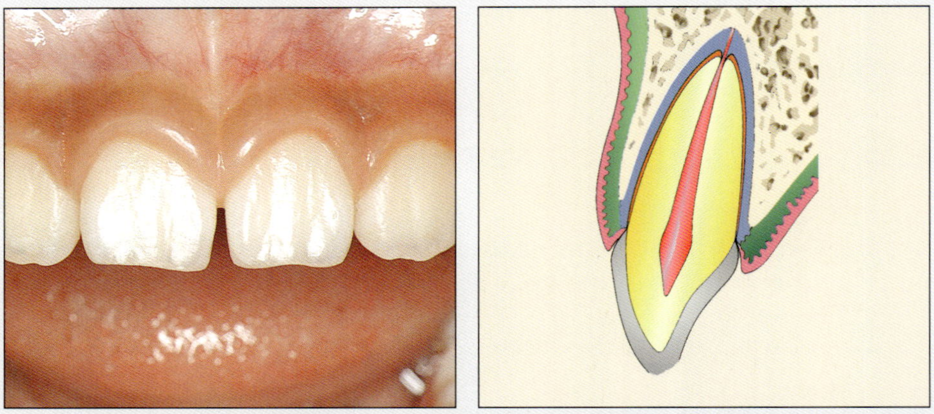

Figs 3-2c and d After selective grinding.

Fig 3-3 Treatment of uncomplicated crown fracture (no tooth fragment available)

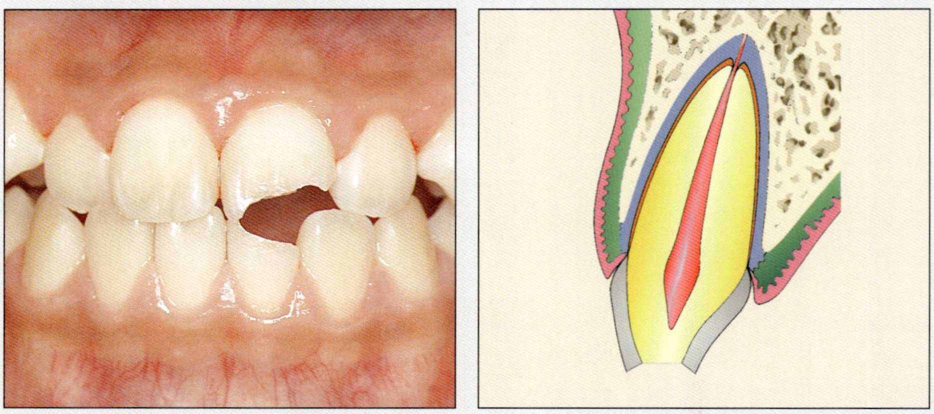

Figs 3-3a and b Preoperative view.

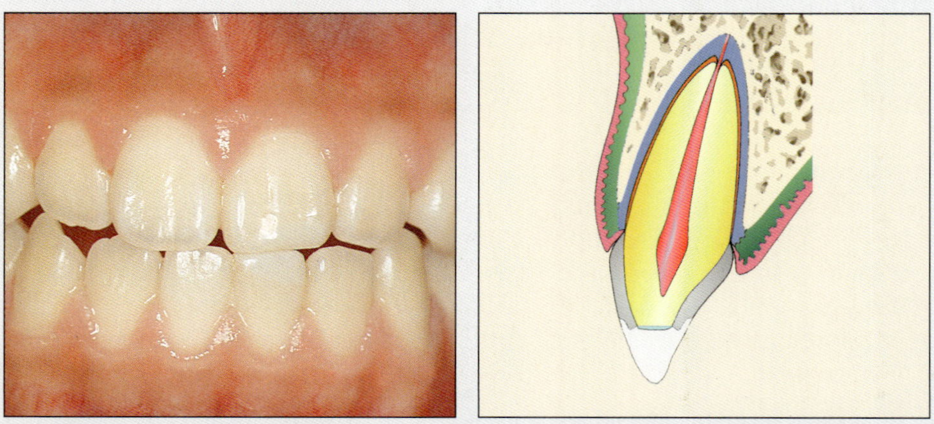

Figs 3-3c and d After restorative treatment with composite resin.

Fig 3-4 Treatment of uncomplicated crown fracture (tooth fragment has been saved)

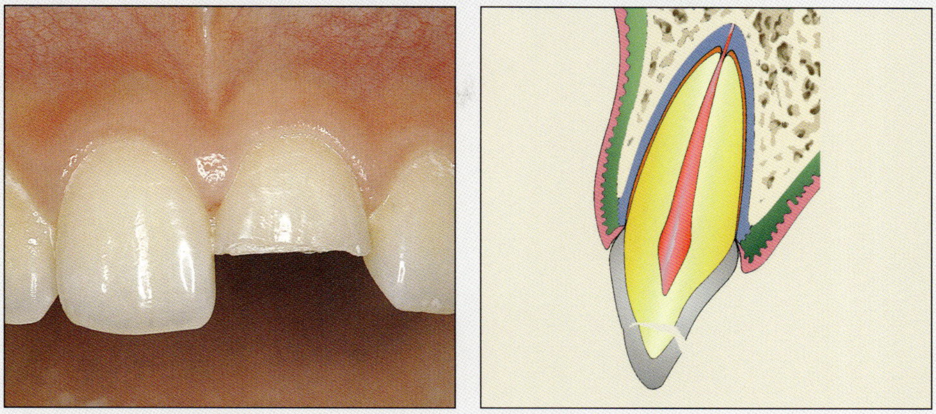

Figs 3-4a and b Preoperative view.

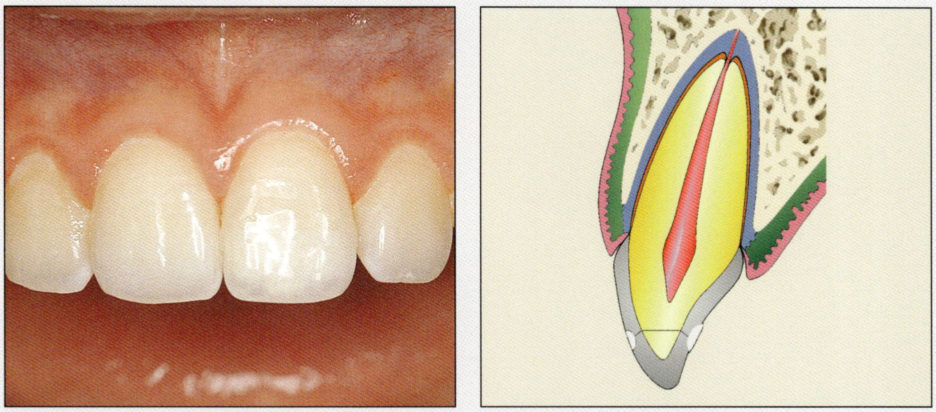

Figs 3-4c and d After reattachment of the tooth fragment.

Fig 3-5 Treatment of complicated crown fracture with minimal pulp exposure (tooth fragment available)

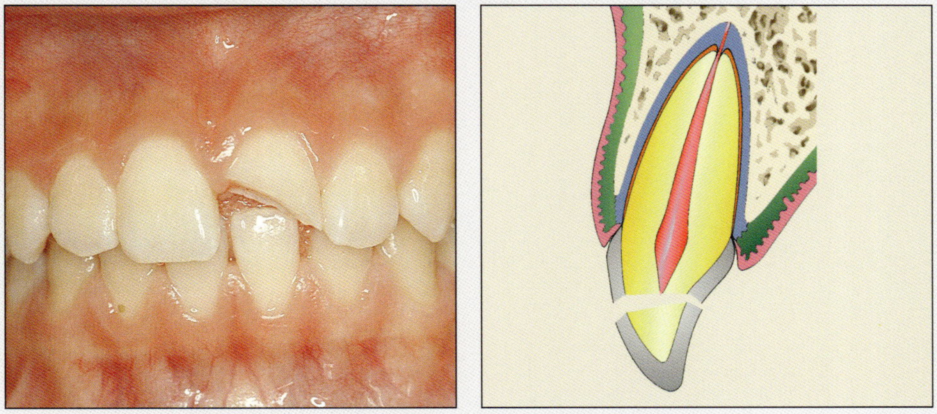

Figs 3-5a and b Preoperative view.

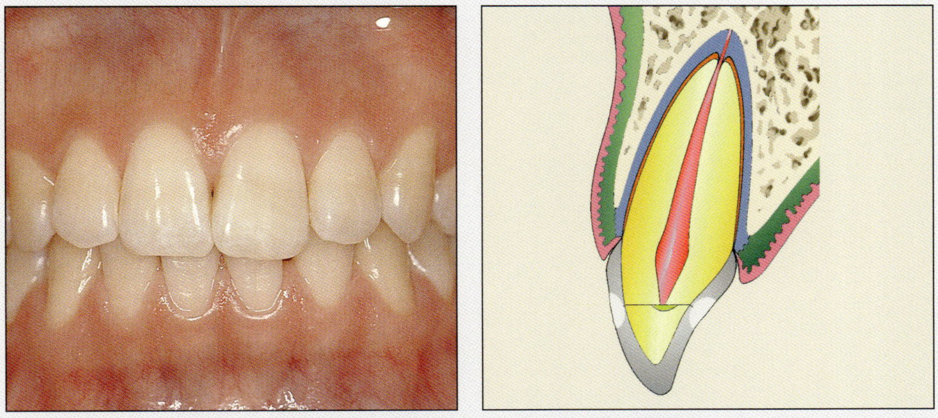

Figs 3-5c and d After pulp capping and reattachment of the tooth fragment.

Fig 3-6 Treatment of complicated crown fracture with considerable pulp exposure (tooth fragment available)

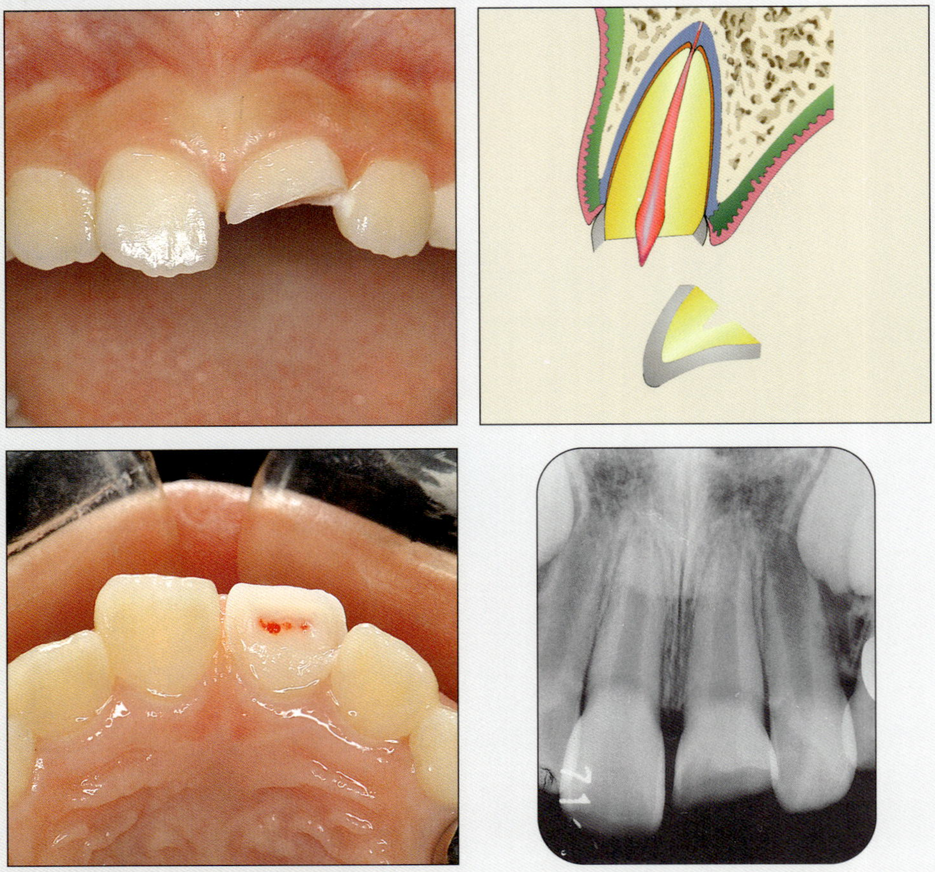

Figs 3-6a to d Preoperative views. Note that the tooth has an incompletely formed root.

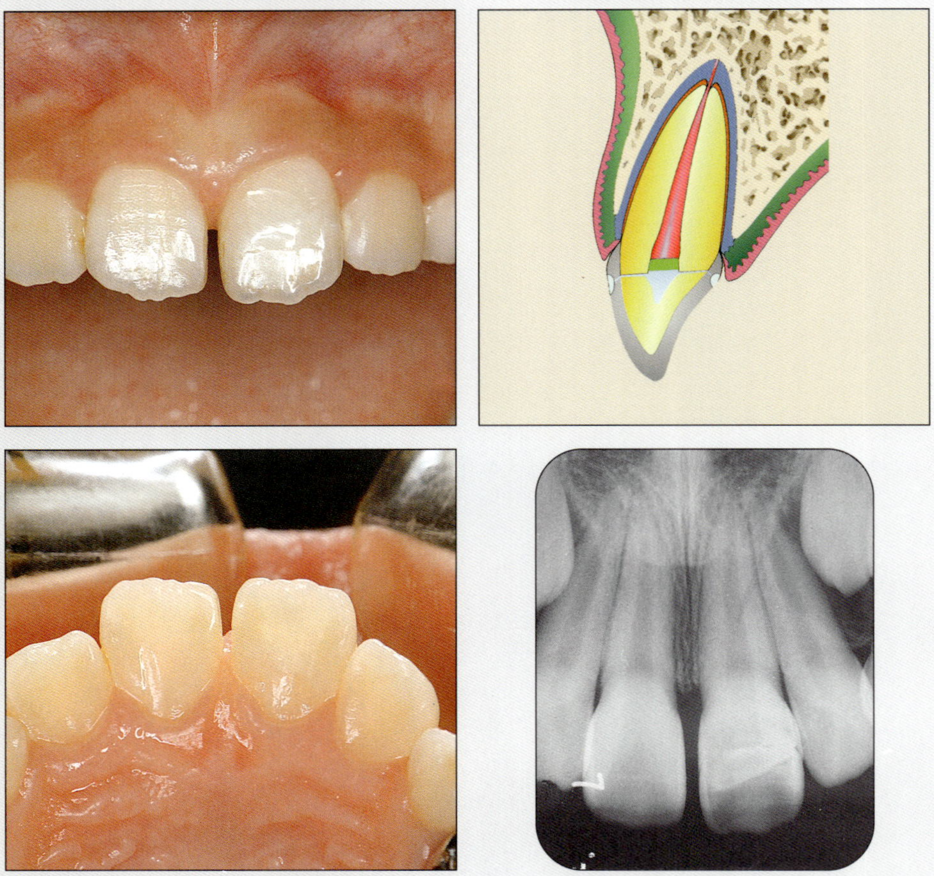

Figs 3-6e to h After partial pulpotomy and reattachment of the tooth fragment. Root formation is almost complete after 1 year and 4 months.

Fig 3-7 Treatment of crown fracture combined with luxation injury (tooth fragments available)

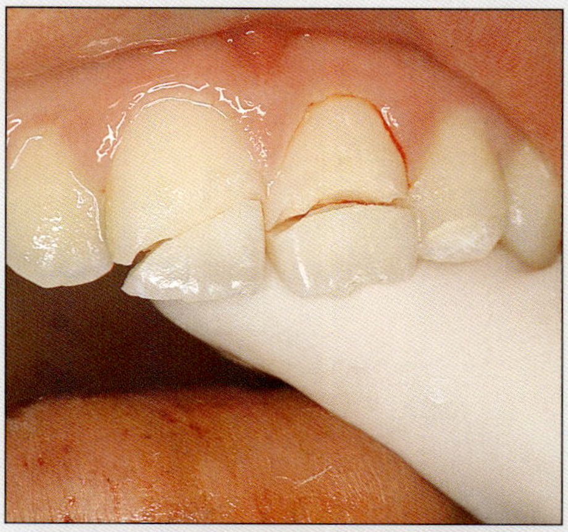

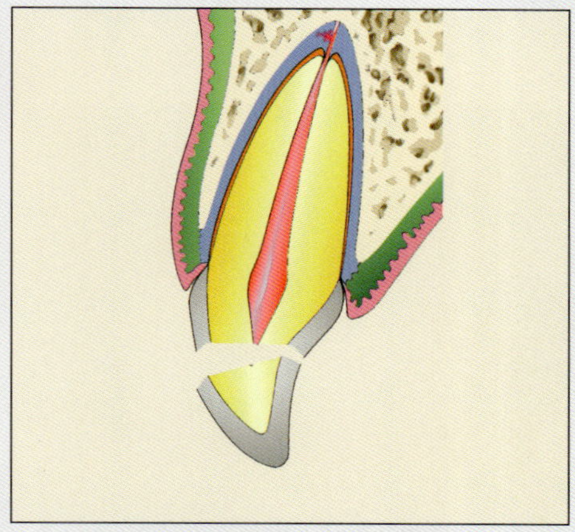

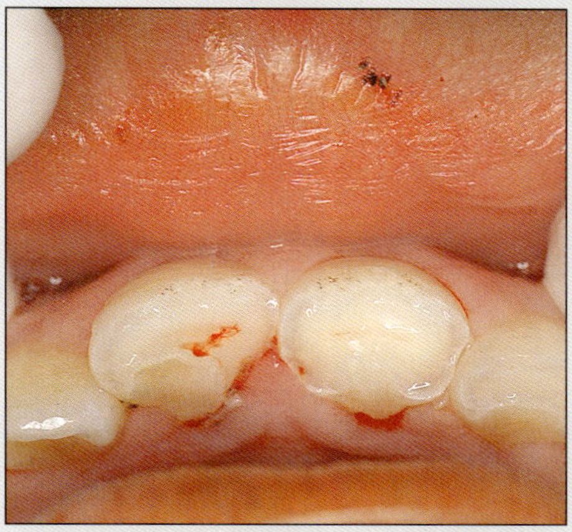

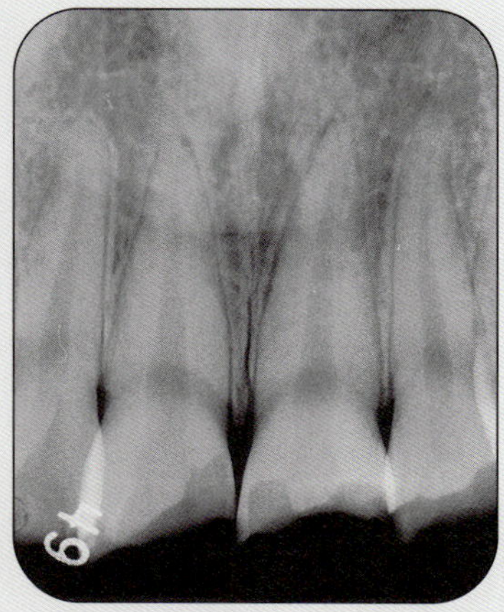

Figs 3-7a to d Preoperative views. Note crown fractures of teeth 8, 9, and 10. Only tooth 9 had no response to EPT.

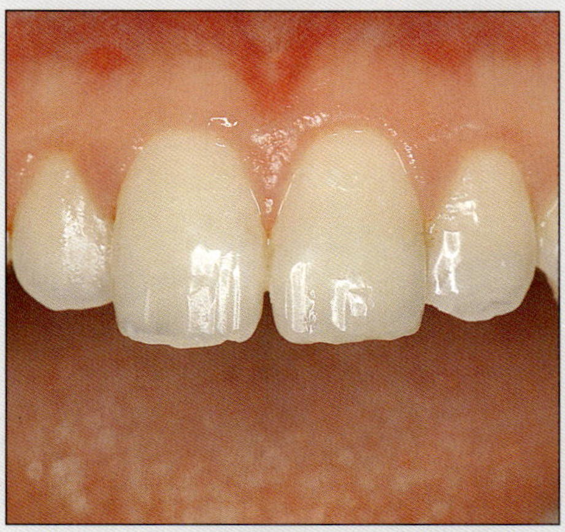

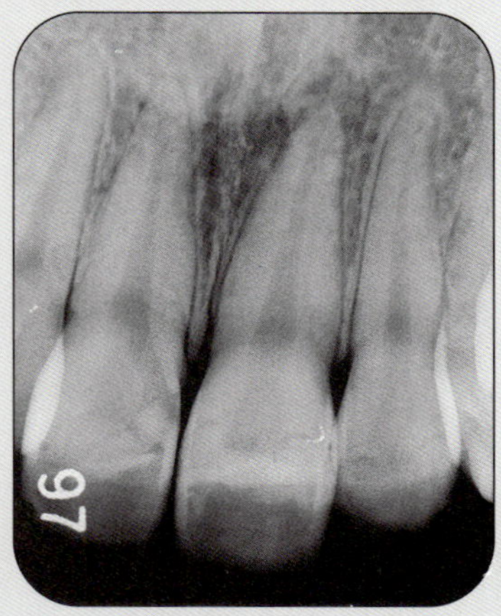

Fig 3-7e After restorative treatment.

Fig 3-7f Three months later, tooth 9 has considerable percussion pain; therefore, necrosis of the pulp is suspected.

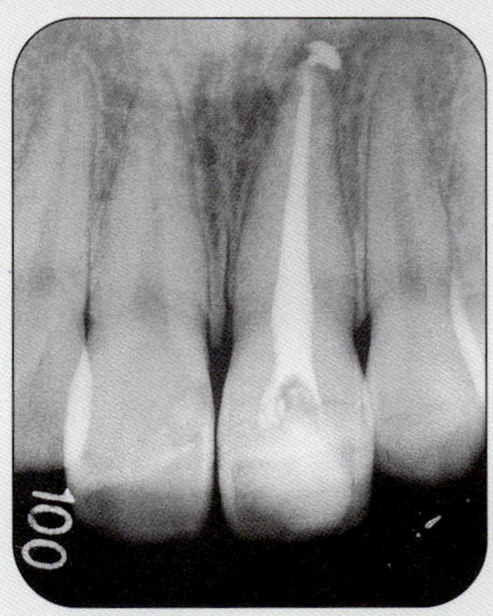

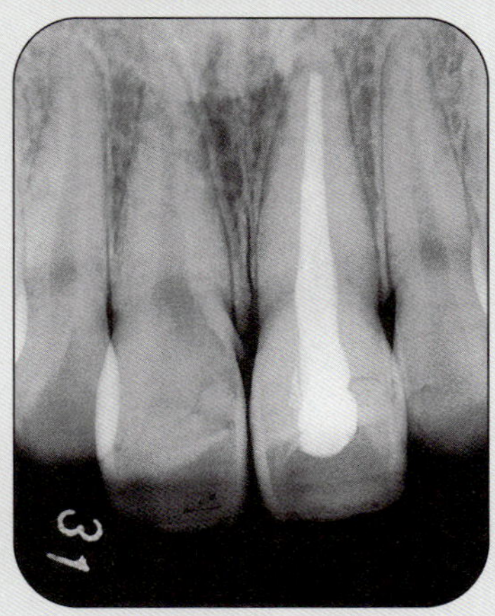

Fig 3-7g Apexification using calcium hydroxide.

Fig 3-7h Nine months later, the root canal treatment is completed.

Fig 3-8 Treatment of crown fracture with large pulp exposure (tooth fragment available)

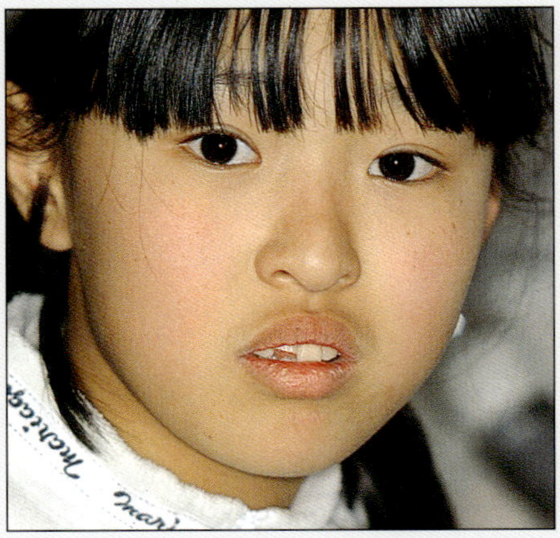
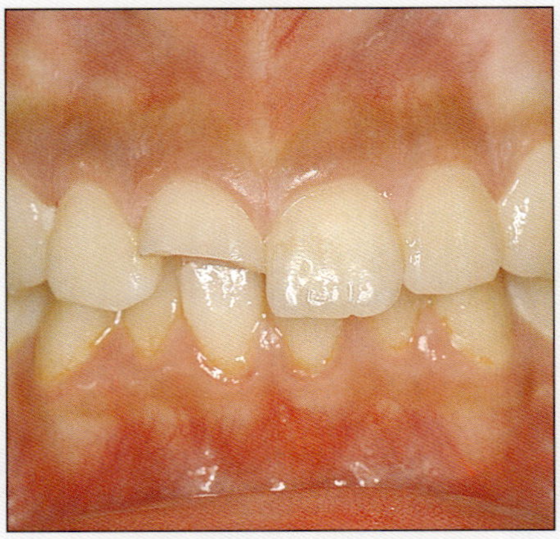
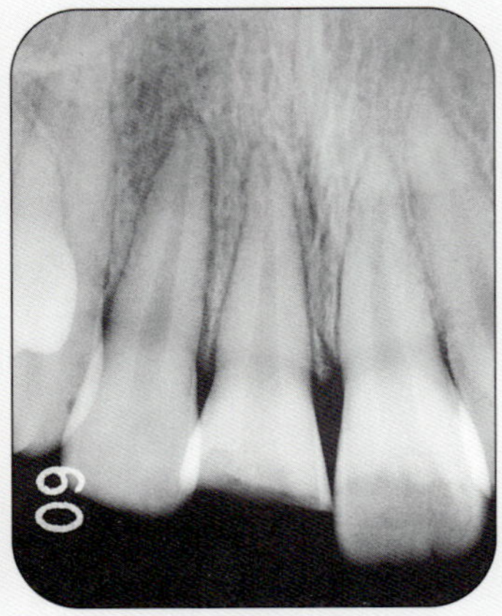

Figs 3-8a to c Preoperative views.

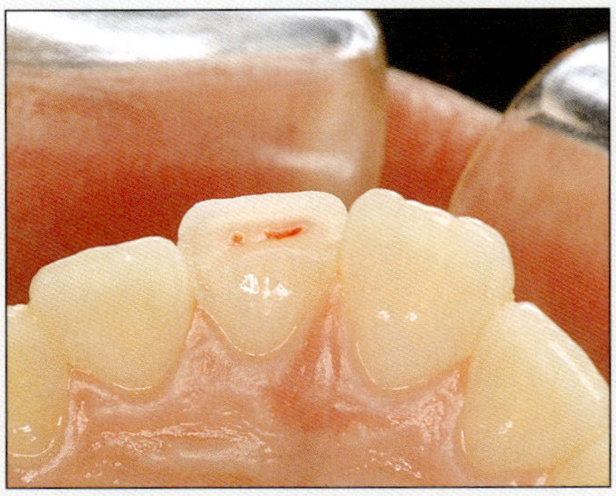

Fig 3-8d Preoperative examination and diagnosis.

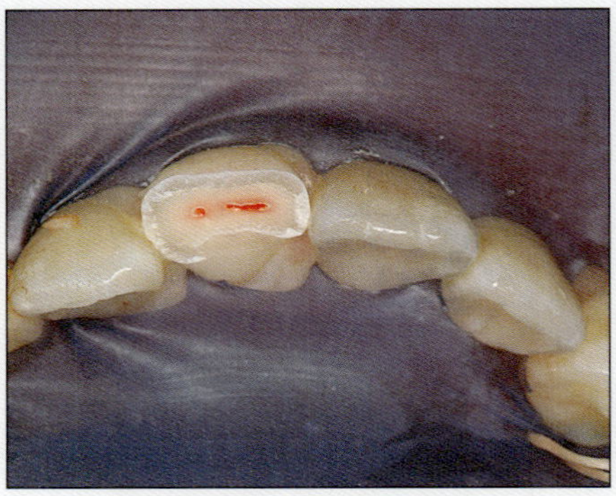

Fig 3-8e Anesthesic and rubber dam applied.

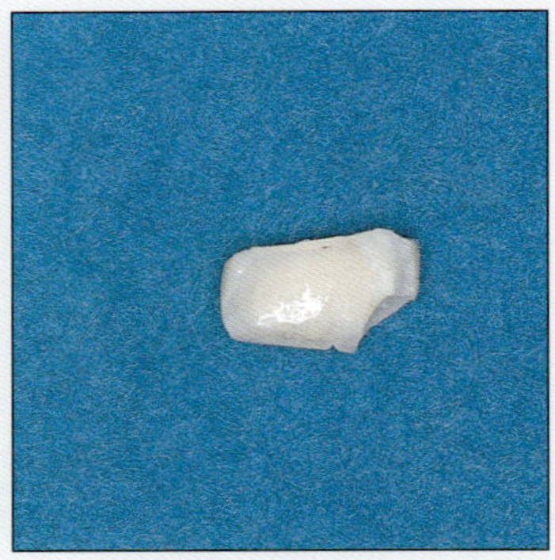

Fig 3-8f Examination of tooth fragment.

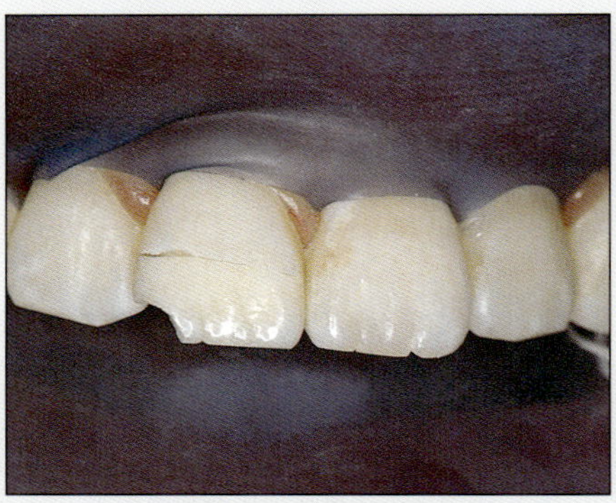

Fig 3-8g Fit of the tooth fragment and remaining tooth is checked.

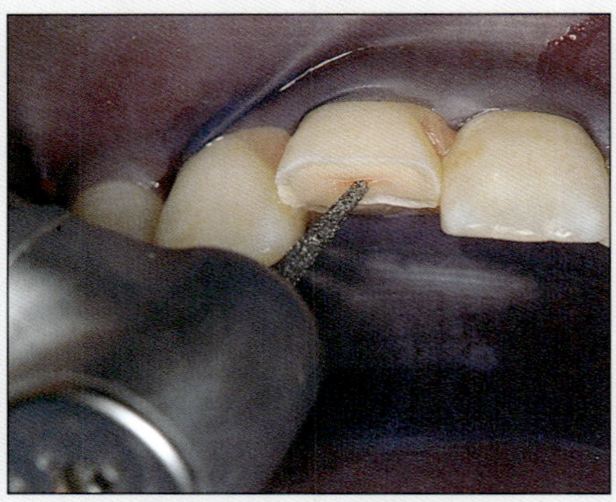

Fig 3-8h Partial pulpotomy.

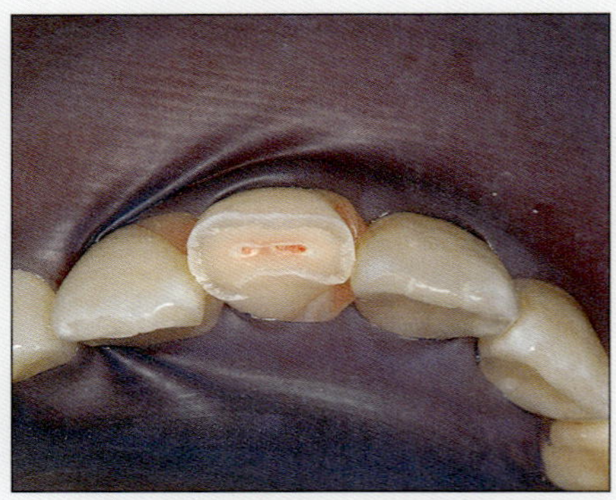

Fig 3-8i After rinsing and hemostasis.

Treatment Procedures

The following describes specific procedures for crown fractures such as those with large pulp exposure (Fig 3-8).

1. *Examination and diagnosis*: Radiographs, intraoral photographs, and EPT reveal enamel-dentin fracture with pulp exposure (Figs 3-8a to d).
2. *Pretreatment preparation*: Administer local anesthetic and isolate with a rubber dam (Fig 3-8e).

Fig 3-8 (continued)

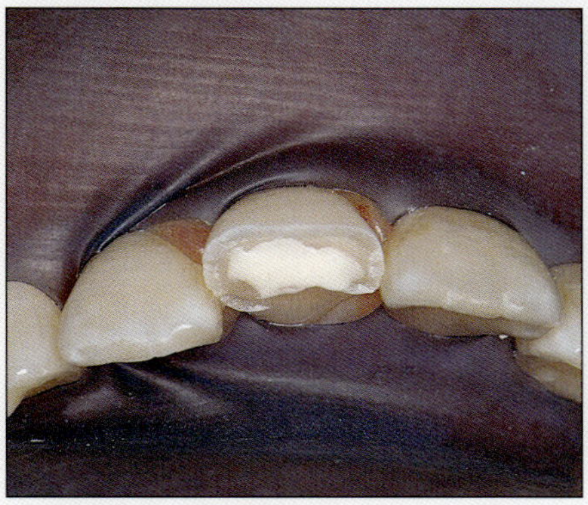

Fig 3-8j After placement of pulp dressing (composite resin).

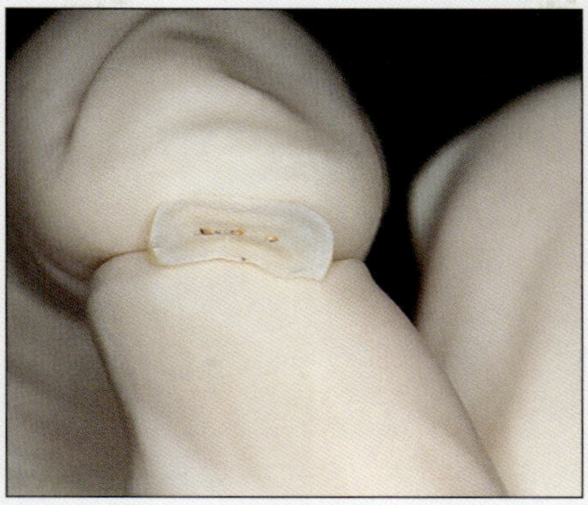

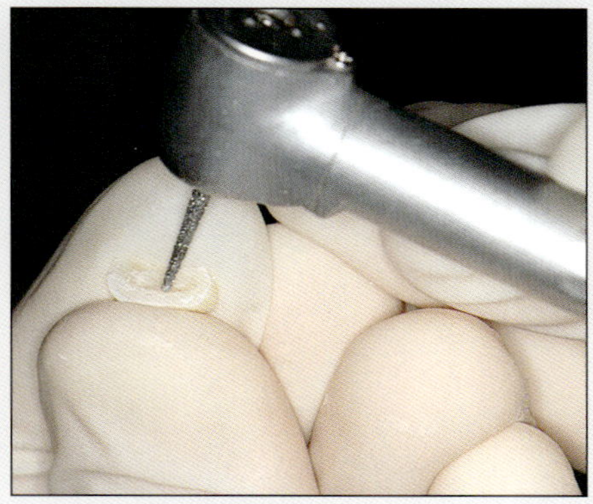

Figs 3-8k and l Removal of pulp tissue from the tooth fragment.

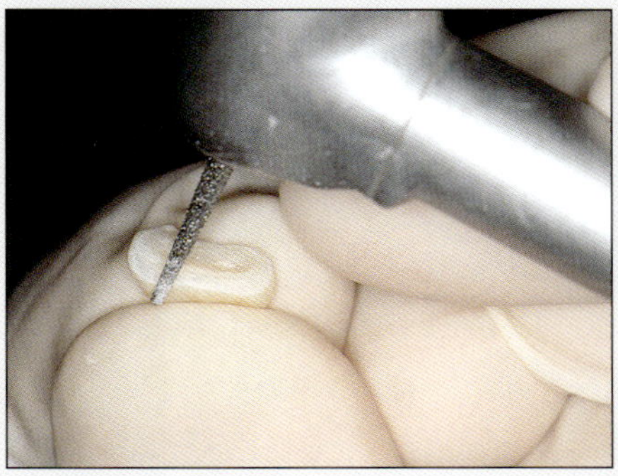

Fig 3-8m Beveling of the tooth fragment.

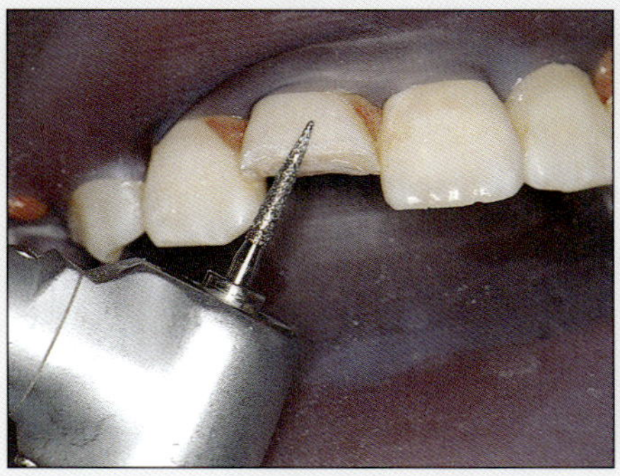

Fig 3-8n Beveling of the original tooth.

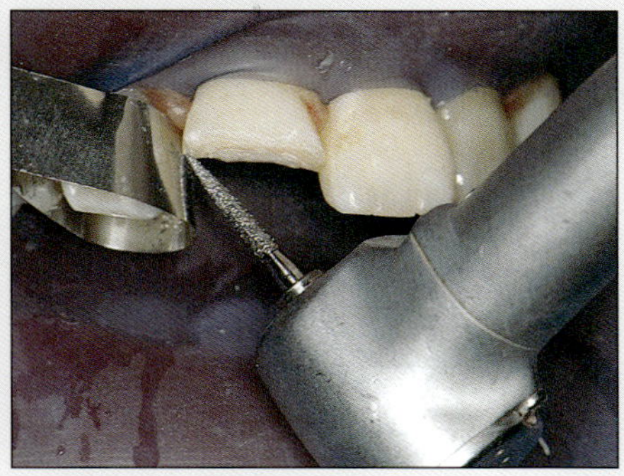

Fig 3-8o Beveling of the proximal surface while protecting the adjacent teeth with metal matrix.

3. *Confirmation of fit of the tooth fragment*: Confirm the fit of the tooth fragment to the remaining tooth and check for enamel defects. Check these and other key points on reattachment (Figs 3-8f and g).
4. *Partial pulpotomy*: Perform partial pulpotomy to remove exposed pulp tissue near the tooth fracture and to leave space for pulpal dressing. Remove 1 to 2 mm of the exposed pulp tissue under a water spray with a new, sterilized diamond bur in a high-speed handpiece (Fig 3-8h).
5. *Cleansing and hemostasis of the amputated pulp surface*: Alternate cleansing with sodium hypochlorite and 3% hydrogen peroxide (Fig 3-8i).
6. *Pulp dressing*: Use a calcium hydroxide cement or composite resin for pulp dressing (Fig 3-8j).
7. *Preparation of the tooth fragment*: Remove any remaining pulp tissue from the pulp horns of the tooth fragment (Figs 3-8k and l). Then bevel the entire periphery of the fractured surface (Fig 3-8m).
8. *Beveling the remaining tooth*: Bevel the entire periphery of the fractured surface of the remaining tooth. Reattachment of the tooth fragments depends on the adhesive strength to enamel. Enamel fracture usually occurs parallel to the enamel rods; therefore, it is difficult to enhance adhesive strength by etching. Provide a bevel to use as much of the adhesive surface as possible (which is at a right angle to the enamel rods) (Figs 3-8n and o).

Fig 3-8 (continued)

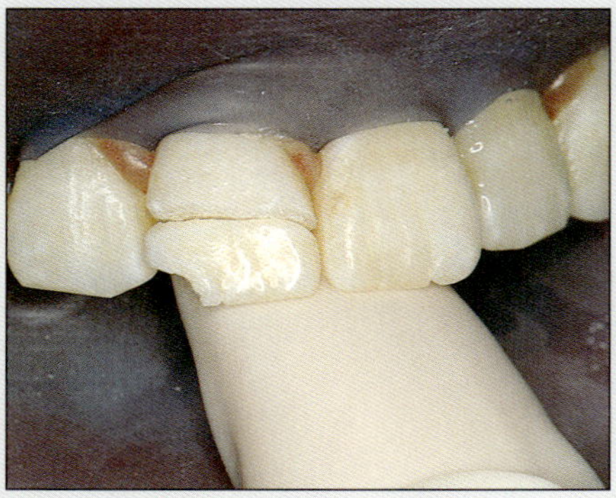

Fig 3-8p Try-in of tooth fragment.

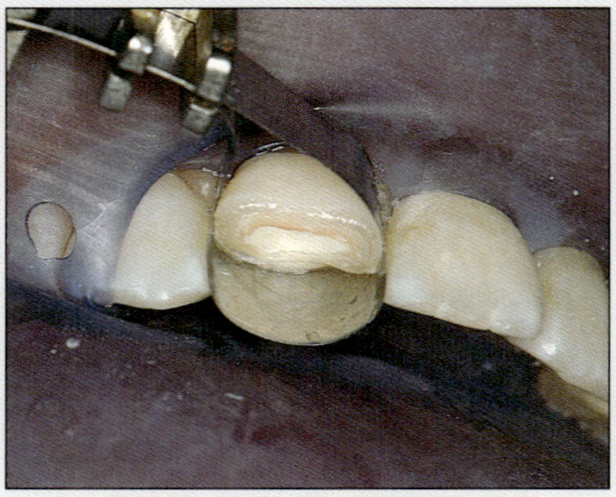

Fig 3-8q Fitting the Tofflemire retainer and metal matrix band.

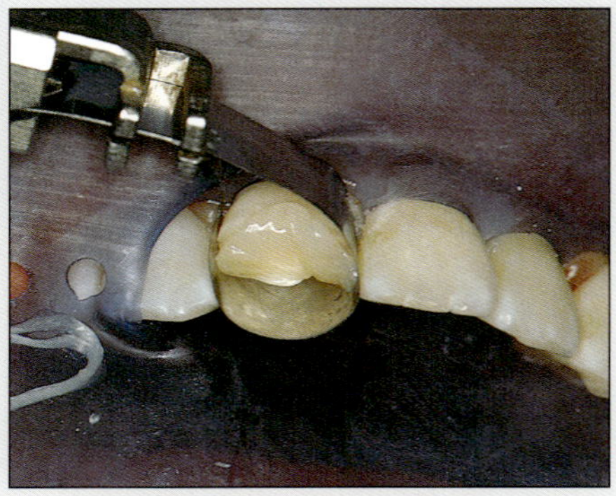

Fig 3-8r Etching and bonding before application of the composite resin on the fractured surface.

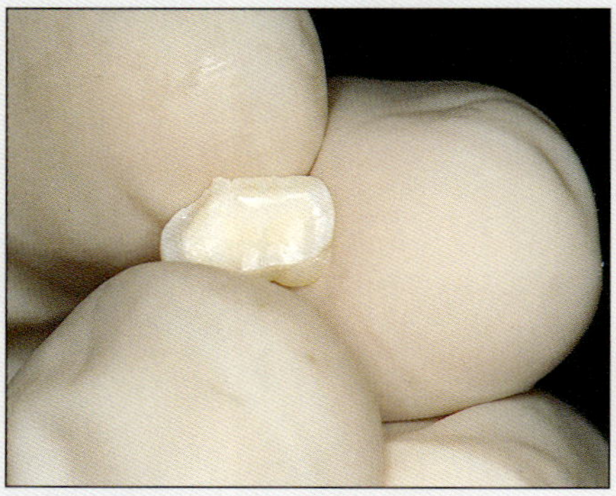

Fig 3-8s

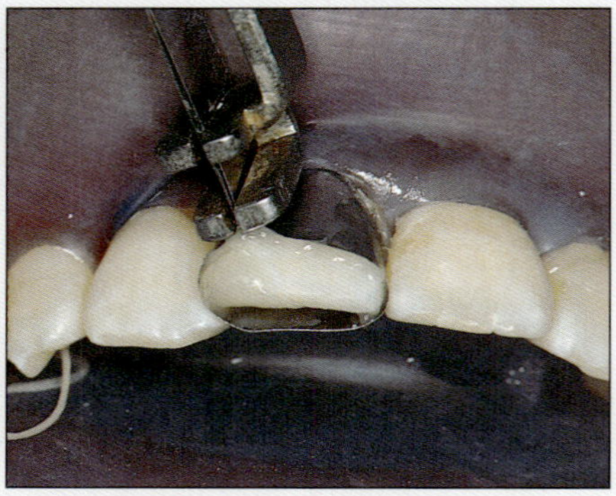

Fig 3-8t

Fig 3-8s Etching and bonding of the tooth fragment is followed by the application of composite resin to the fractured surface.

Fig 3-8t Fitting the tooth fragment to the tooth and tightening the matrix band. Excess composite resin is removed before application of composite resin to the remaining enamel defect. Reshaping and light curing follow.

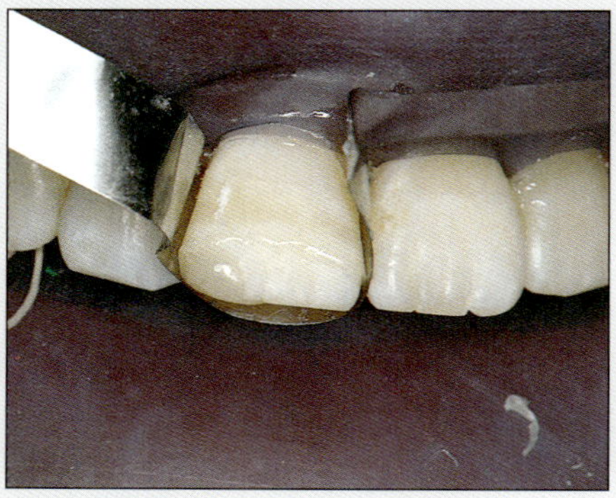

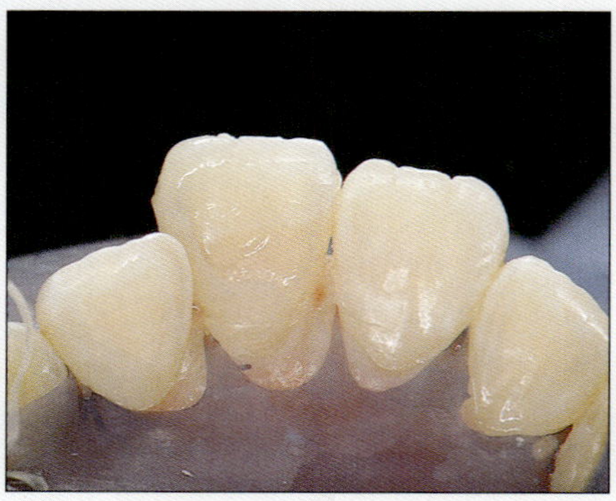

Figs 3-8u and v After the removal of the matrix band.

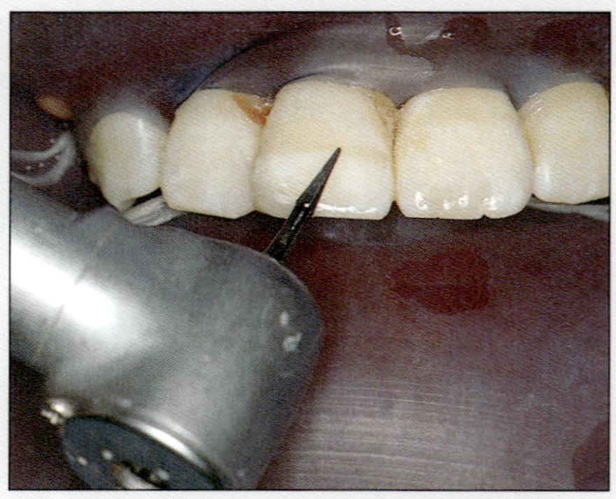

Fig 3-8w Polishing and reshaping with a finishing bur.

9. *Try-in of the tooth fragment*: Confirm the position and direction of the tooth fragment for reattachment (Fig 3-8p).
10. *Fitting the Tofflemire retainer and metal matrix band*: Use the matrix band for reattachment. The Tofflemire retainer and the Universal metal matrix band are used to accurately reposition the tooth fragment to the remaining tooth (Fig 3-8q).
11. *Etching and bonding*: Apply etchant and bonding agent to both the original tooth and the tooth fragment as recommended by the manufacturer of the materials used.

Fig 3-8 (continued)

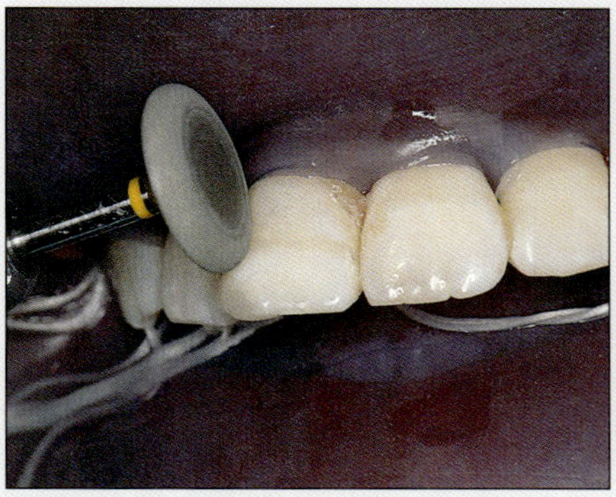

Fig 3-8x Polishing and reshaping with a white silicone point.

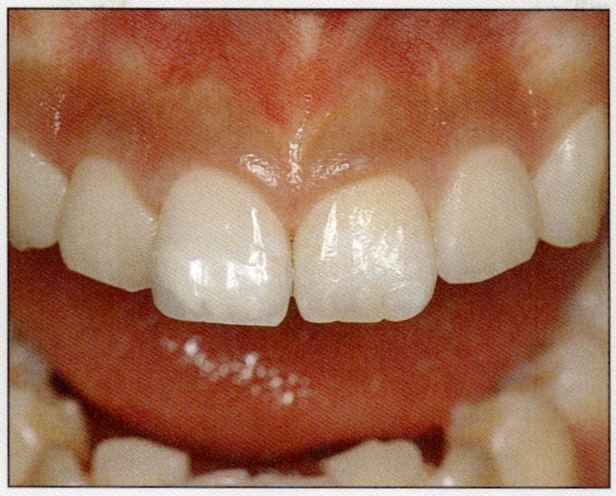

Fig 3-8y

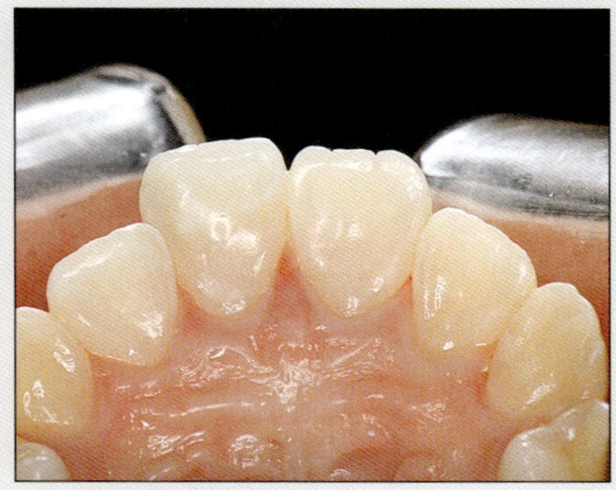

Fig 3-8z

Figs 3-8y to bb Postoperative views.

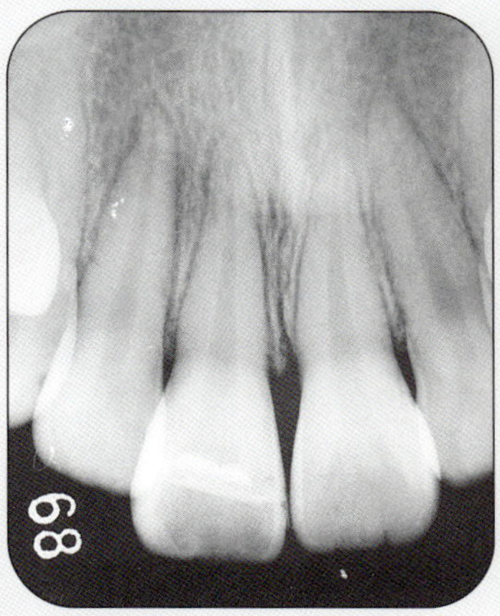

Fig 3-8aa

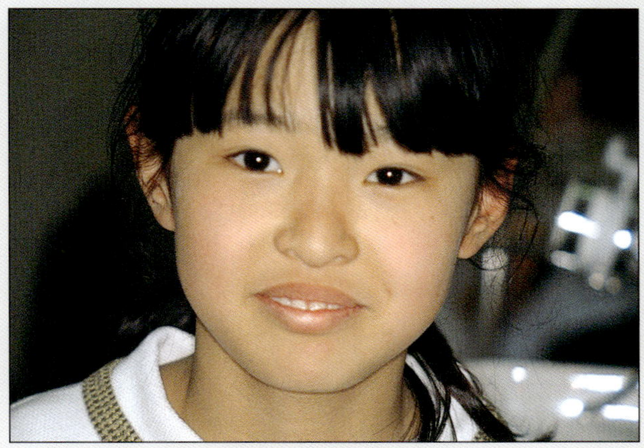

Fig 3-8bb

12. *Composite resin application*: Apply light-cured composite resin to the remaining tooth and the tooth fragment (Figs 3-8r and s).
13. *Attaching the tooth fragment to the remaining tooth*: After closely adapting the fractured surfaces with composite resin, tighten the retainer (Fig 3-8t). By doing this, the tooth fragment is naturally repositioned mesiodistally and buccolingually. Be careful, however, not to extrude the tooth fragment coronally. Remove excess composite resin and restore any enamel defects, then light cure for 40 seconds from the incisal edge.
14. *Removal of the matrix, reshaping, and polishing*: Using a polishing carbide bur and white silicone point, remove the excess composite resin, and reshape and polish the resin (Figs 3-8u to x).
15. *Follow-up*: Examine after 1 week, 1 month, and 3 months. Check for discomfort and possible pulp necrosis, and evaluate esthetics (Figs 3-8y to bb).

If pulp capping is not necessary, omit steps 4, 5, and 6.

Fig 3-9 Restorative treatment with composite resin

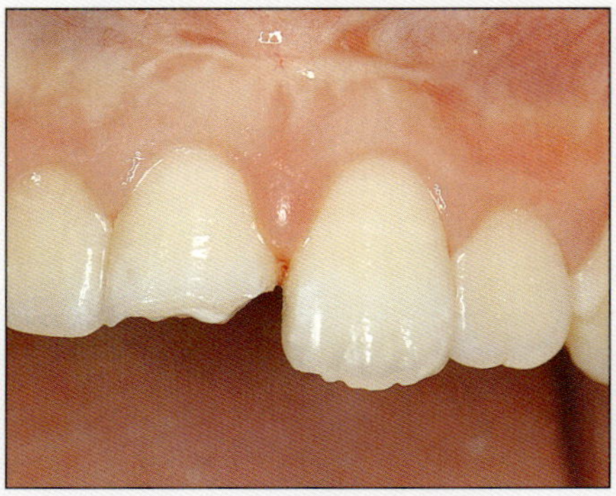

Fig 3-9a Preoperative view.

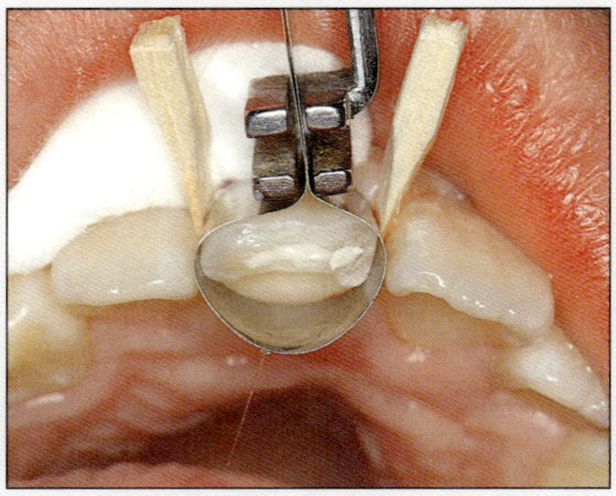

Fig 3-9b After cleansing the tooth surface, pulp capping, beveling, and fitting the matrix band.

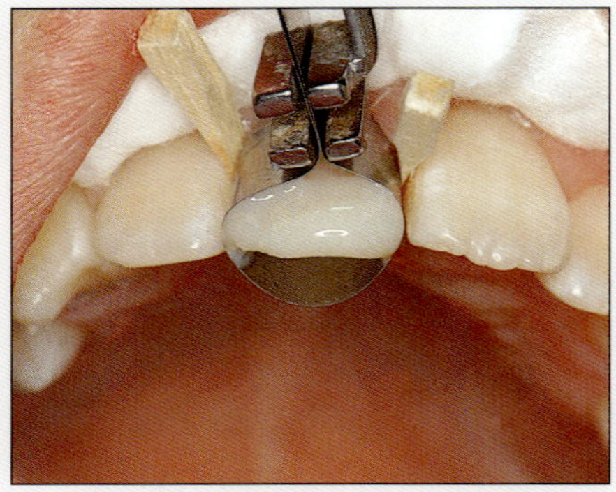

Fig 3-9c Composite resin is applied and shaped.

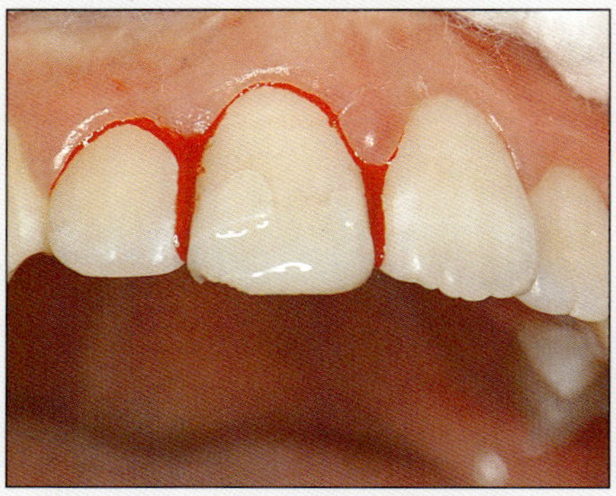

Fig 3-9d After curing of the composite resin.

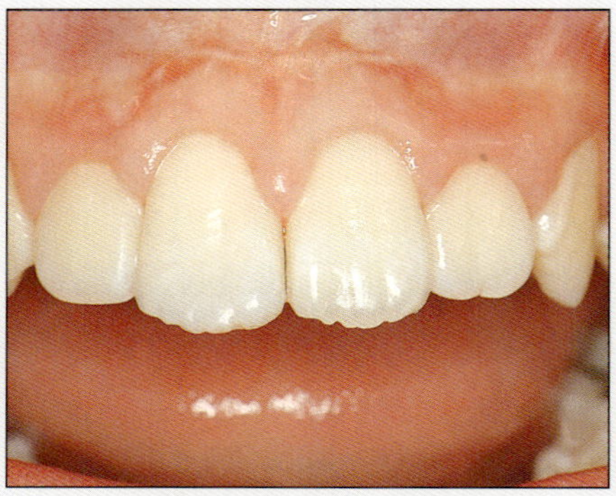

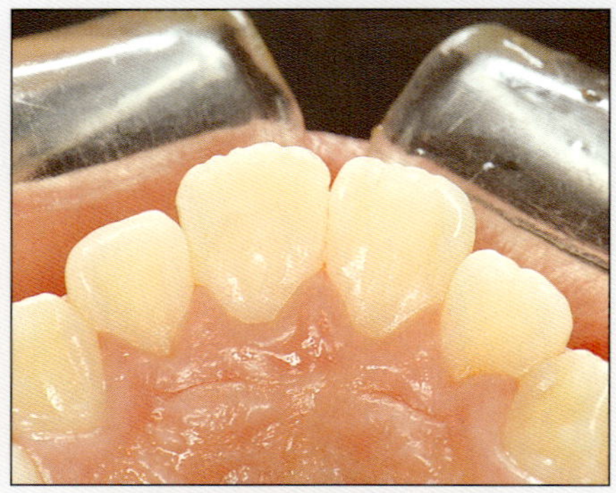

Figs 3-9e and f Composite resin is reshaped and polished.

Where there is no tooth fragment available, the original tooth is beveled, the metal matrix is fit, and the etchant and the bonding agent are applied. The tooth is restored using composite resin only (Fig 3-9).

Even when pulp necrosis is suspected, restorative treatment as described should be performed. Apexification can be performed later (see Chapter 6, luxations section). A diagnosis of pulp necrosis cannot be made immediately in a traumatized tooth with an immature root.

It may seem to be a misdirected effort to restore an immature tooth before completion of endodontic treatment. Procedures such as apexification, however, can take considerable time, and until treatment is finished and the apex has closed, the tooth should be restored to normal function and esthetics as much as possible. After endodontic treatment, a new restoration may be required, but in the meantime the patient has had the use of a reasonably normal tooth (see Fig 3-7).

For adults with fully formed roots, it is best to complete endodontic treatment before beginning restorative treatment.

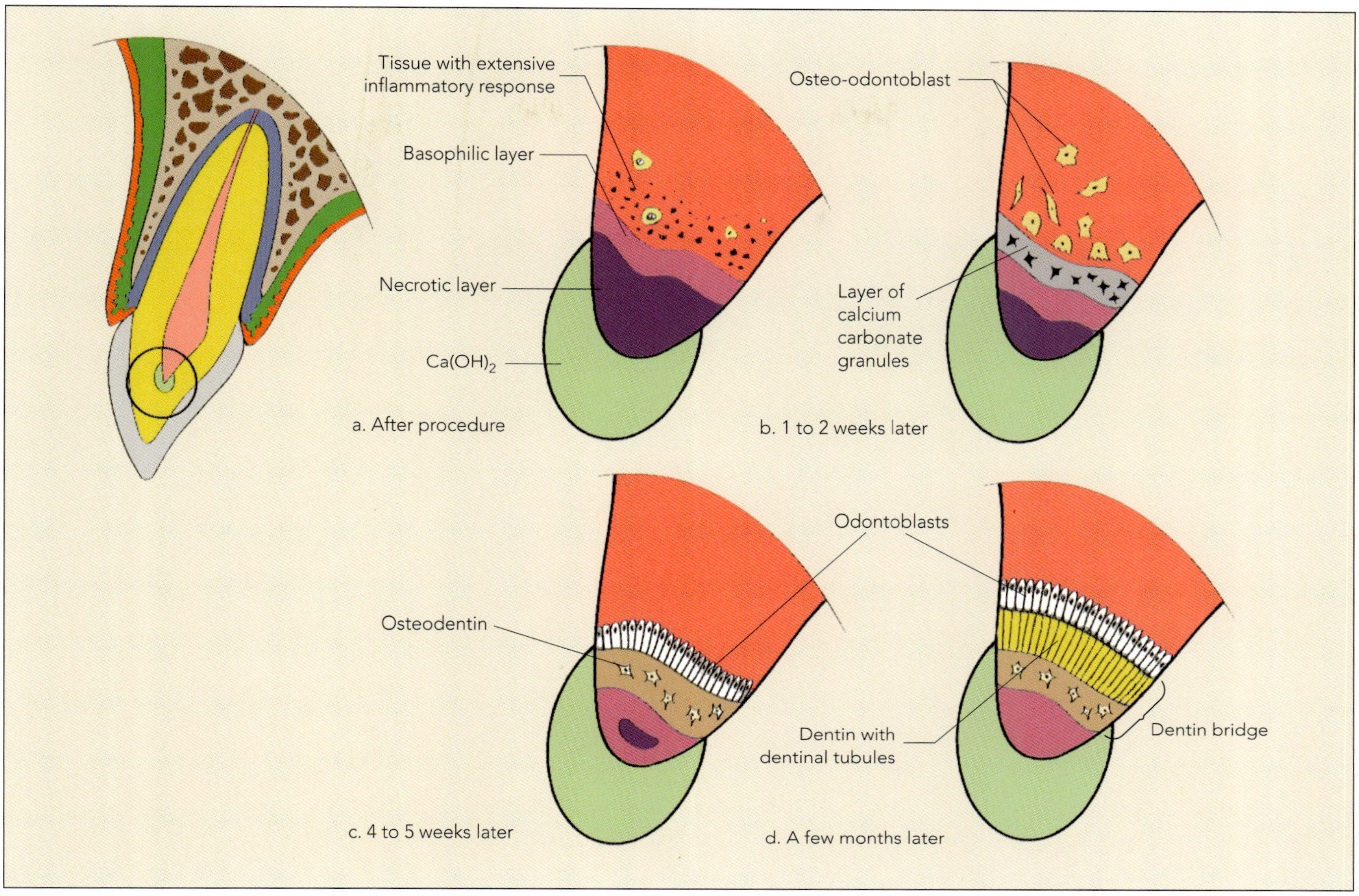

Fig 3-10 Direct pulp capping and formation of dentin bridge.[19-22]

Pulp Capping and Pulp Healing

The pulp-dentin complex is a recognized concept.[9] Generally speaking, dentin exposure means microscopic pulp exposure. As in the case of obvious pulp exposure, a pulp capping procedure should be followed. There are two methods of pulp capping. One is biologic closure of the dentinal tubules and the exposed pulp by accelerating apposition of the tertiary dentin (reparative dentin) by the pulp. A calcium hydroxide preparation is used for this purpose.[10,11] The other method is the physical closure of the exposed pulp or tubules with dentin adhesive material. The dentin adhesive resin that forms the resinous infiltrated layer is used for this purpose.[12-18] If the dentin adhesive resin is used for direct pulp capping, not only is microbial invasion and mechanical stimulation prevented, but a dentin bridge is formed on the exposed pulp because of a physical closure of the exposed pulp. The result is the same as direct pulp capping with a calcium hydroxide preparation.[14-16]

Figure 3-10 describes the mechanism of dentin bridge formation (direct pulp capping using calcium hydroxide).

The mechanism of dentin bridge formation[19-22]

1. *Immediately after vital pulp treatment*: A necrotic layer is observed below the calcium hydroxide. The inflammatory tissue response is observed under the necrotic layer (Fig 3-10a).

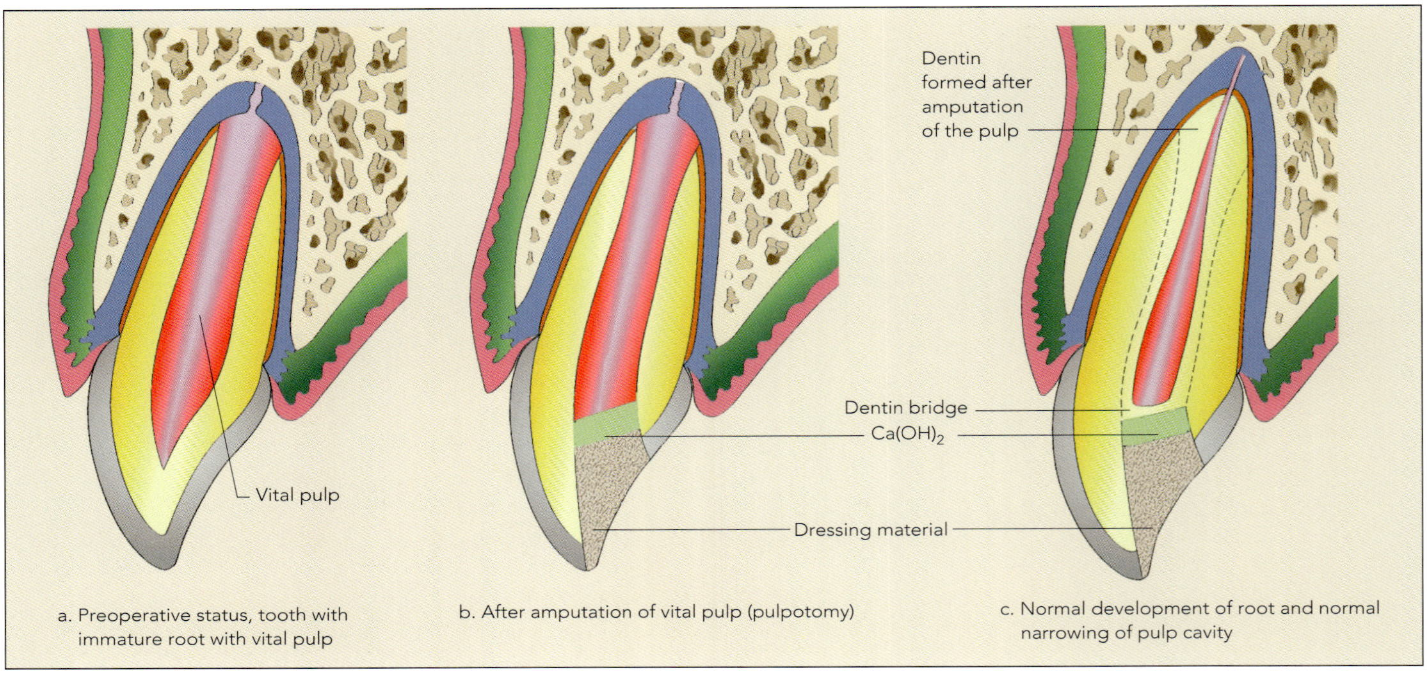

Fig 3-11 Apexogenesis.

2. *After 1 to 2 weeks*: There is a layer with a noticeable deposit of calcium carbonate granules. Beneath that layer, osteo-odontoblasts derived from pulp cells emerge (Fig 3-10b).
3. *After 4 to 5 weeks*: The osteodentin is formed by osteo-odontoblasts, and beneath the osteodentin are odontoblasts (derived from the pulp). Perhaps osteodentin stimulates the arrangement of odontoblasts (Fig 3-10c).
4. *A few months later (final stage)*: The dentin bridge is formed. It is composed of two layers of hard tissue, osteodentin and dentin with dentinal tubules (Fig 3-10d).

These time periods are approximate; variations occur. If the amputation of the pulp in a tooth with an immature root is successfully performed, the remaining pulp tissue is saved and normal narrowing of the pulp cavity and normal development of the root will occur. This normal development of the root observed after the amputation of the pulp of a tooth with an immature root is called ***apexogenesis***[23] (Fig 3-11).

4

Crown-Root Fracture

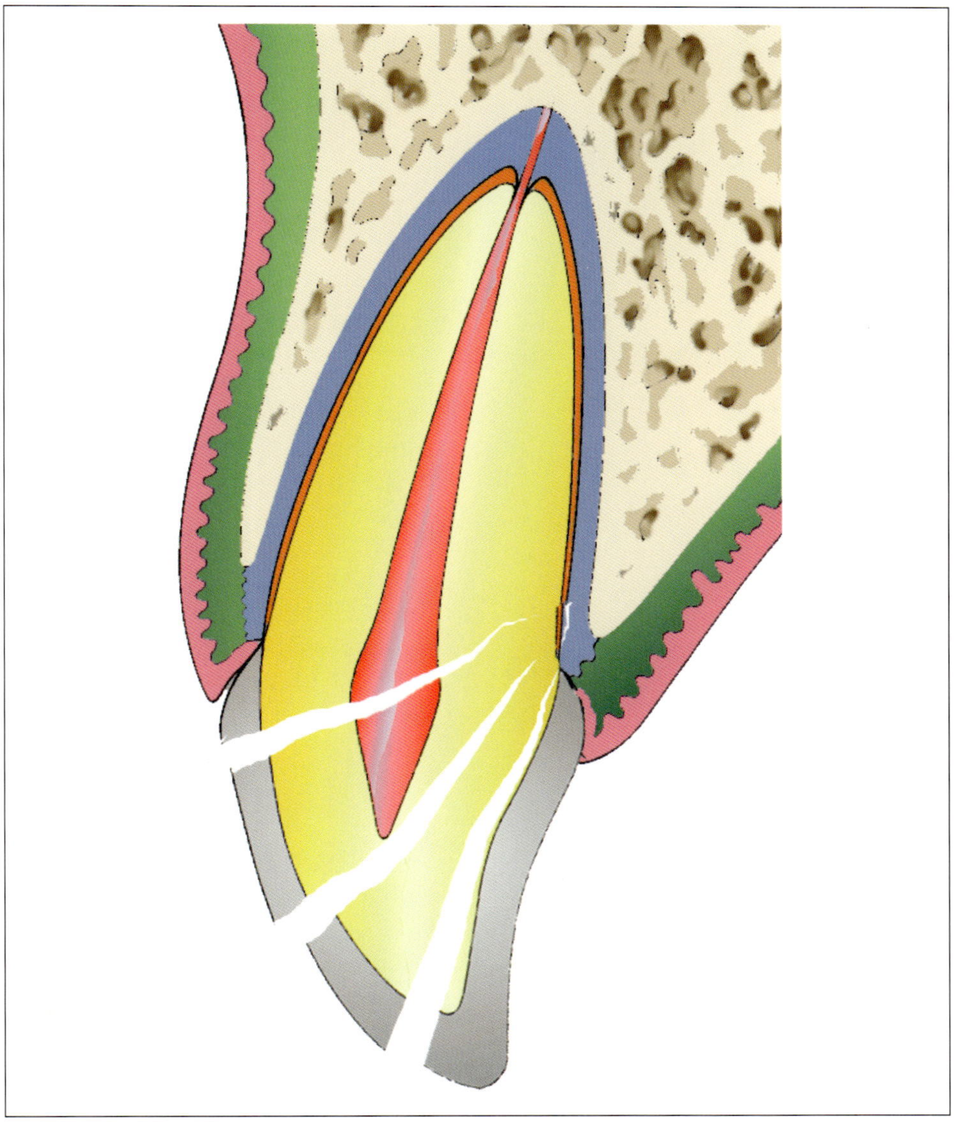

Crown-root fractures are complicated by the extent of injuries. The fractures may be such that the crown and part of the root are shattered into small fragments, or the fracture may be of the chisel-type, in which part of the crown and part of the root fracture remain a single unit. The fractured part of the root is often still attached to the periodontal ligament (PDL), resulting in the fractured tooth segment being loosely approximated to the tooth. Crown-root fractures often expose the pulp. All of the complexities—pulp exposure and attachment to the PDL—result in considerable pain.

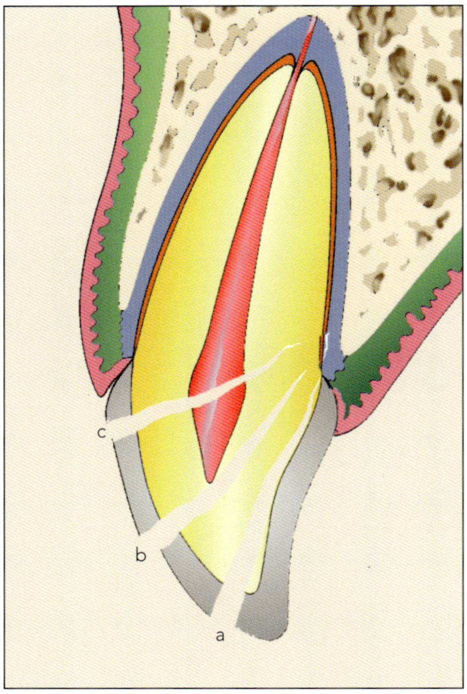

Fig 4-1 Types of crown-root fractures. (a, b) Uncomplicated crown-root fracture. (c) Complicated crown-root fracture.

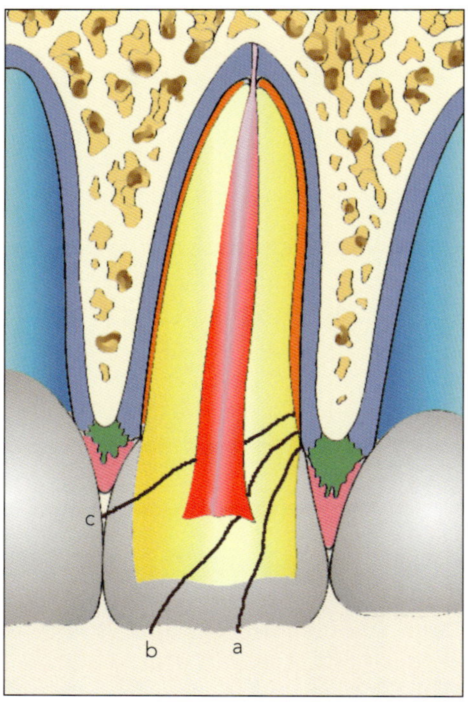

Fig 4-2 Types of crown-root fractures. (a, b) Uncomplicated crown-root fracture. (c) Complicated crown-root fracture.

Description

Uncomplicated crown-root fracture

In uncomplicated fractures, the fracture passes through enamel, dentin, and cementum without pulp exposure. The fracture may be very close to the pulp and perhaps result in a minuscule exposure (Figs 4-1[a and b] and 4-2[a and b]). Usually, the position of the fracture in the cementum is near the crestal bone margin or slightly above. There is no or only slight bleeding from the periodontium.

Complicated crown-root fracture

In complicated fractures, the fracture passes through the enamel, the dentin, and the cementum with pulp exposure (Figs 4-1c and 4-2c). The position of the fracture in the cementum varies from the suprabony margin to the intrabony margin, and there is usually bleeding from the periodontium and the pulp.

Examination and Diagnosis: Key Points

The general characteristic of the crown-root fracture is that the fracture line is observed in the crown and the tooth fragment remains in place despite displacement of the tooth. This is because one part of the tooth fragment remains connected to the alveolar bone or gingiva through the periodontal membrane.

During examination, it is important to check the extent of fracture and the existence of pulp exposure and bleeding by inspection and palpation. It is especially important to note the existence and the degree of bleeding from the periodontium and the pulp because these factors affect the treatment plan. In most cases, there is less bleeding in uncomplicated crown-root fractures and extensive bleeding in complicated crown-root fractures.

Treatment Plan

Uncomplicated crown-root fracture

An attempt should be made to reattach the tooth fragment as described for crown fractures (see Chapter 3, Crown Fracture).

If the pulp is exposed, pulp capping should be performed first. If possible, this is performed while the tooth fragment is attached to the surrounding tissue (Figs 4-3a to f). The tooth fragment needs to be mechanically displaced enough to allow for access to do the pulp capping. If there is no tooth fragment available, restore the tooth with composite resin only.

Complicated crown-root fracture

Because these fractures include pulp exposure, extrusion of the root is often necessary after removal of the tooth fragment to re-establish the biologic width. Restorative treatment is then selected (Figs 4-4a to f).

Fig 4-3 Treatment procedures for uncomplicated crown-root fracture

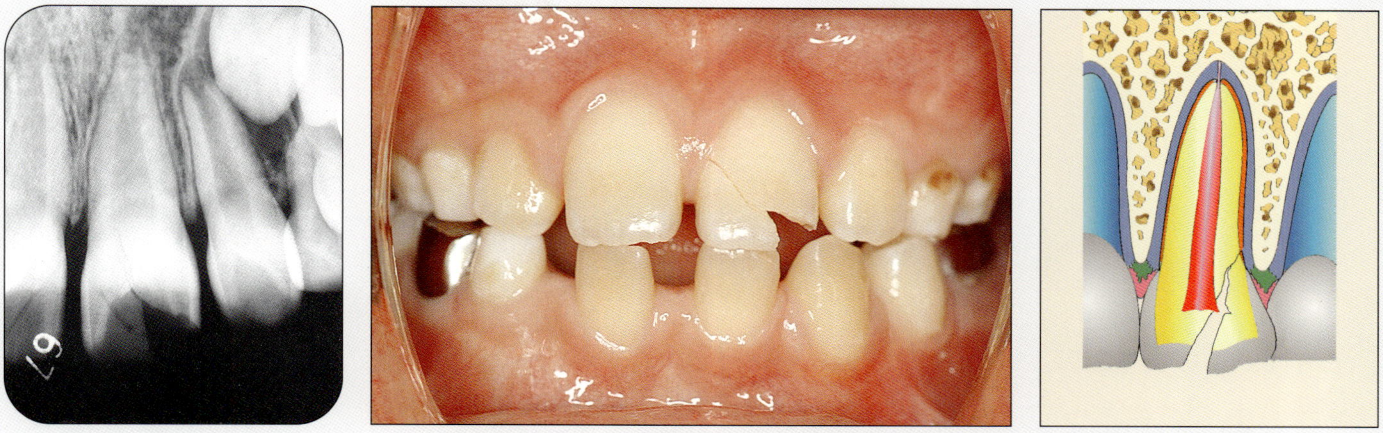

Figs 4-3a to c Preoperative views of injury to an 8-year-old boy.

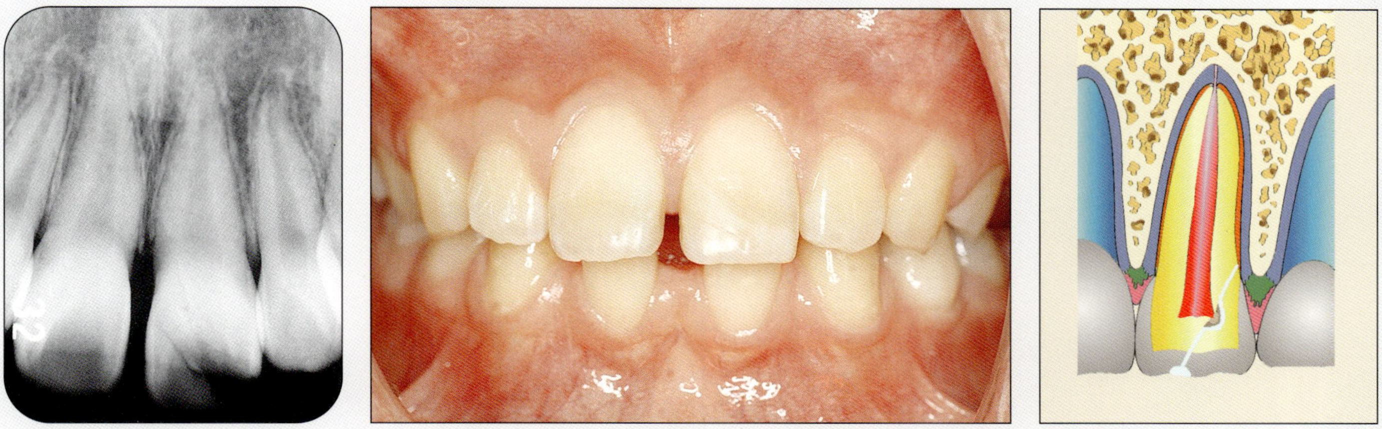

Figs 4-3d to f After reattachment of the tooth fragment.

Treatment Procedures

Uncomplicated crown-root fracture (Fig 4-3)

1. *Examination and diagnosis*: Use radiographs, inspection (including intraoral photographs), palpation, and electric pulp test (EPT) to confirm uncomplicated crown-root fracture (Figs 4-3a and b).
2. *Local anesthesia*: Administer local anesthesic if necessary.
3. *Try-in of the tooth fragment*: Check the fit of the tooth fragment to the tooth and check for any enamel defects. Check the key points on reattachment (Fig 4-3g).
4. *Irrigation of the wound surface*: Use sodium hypochlorite and 3% hydrogen peroxide alternately for irrigation of the fractured surface and for hemostasis of the soft tissues.
5. *Pulp capping*: If there is slight pulp exposure, use calcium hydroxide cement for pulp dressing (Fig 4-3h).
6. *Reattachment of the tooth fragment*: This procedure should be performed while the tooth fragment is connected to the surrounding tissue. Do not remove the tooth fragment from the oral cavity. First, remove any pulp tissue from the pulp horn of the tooth fragment and bevel the entire periphery of the fracture line of the tooth fragment. Next, bevel the entire periphery of the fractured surface of the remain-

Fig 4-3 (Continued)

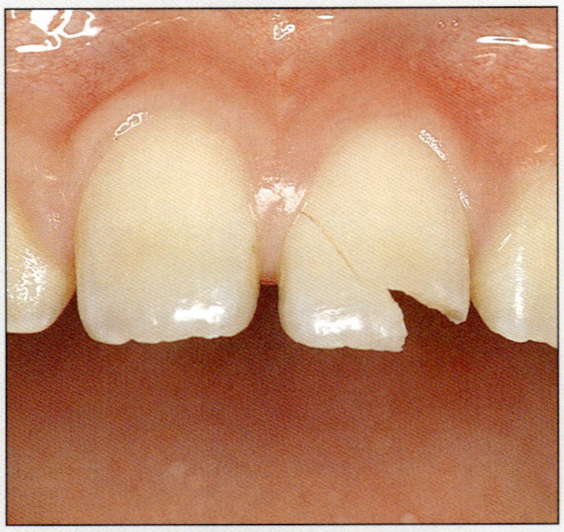

Fig 4-3g The fit of tooth fragment is checked.

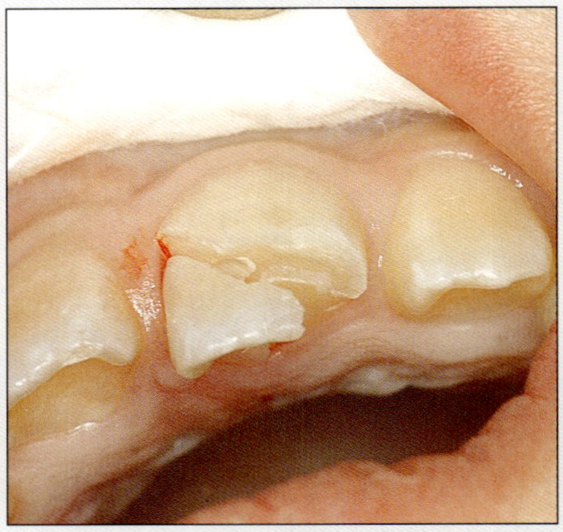

Fig 4-3h The pulp horn is capped.

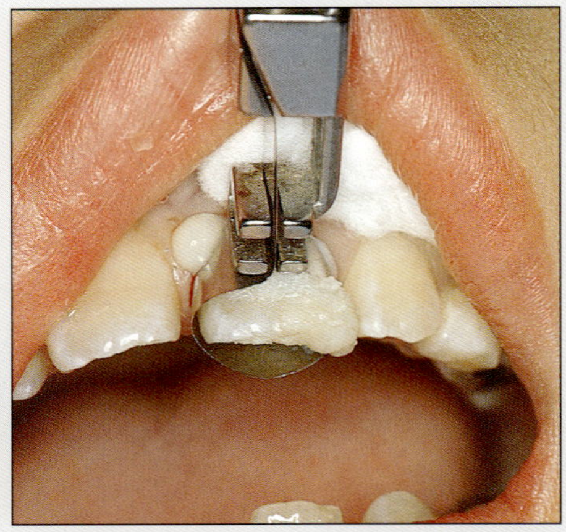

Fig 4-3i The tooth fragment is reattached.

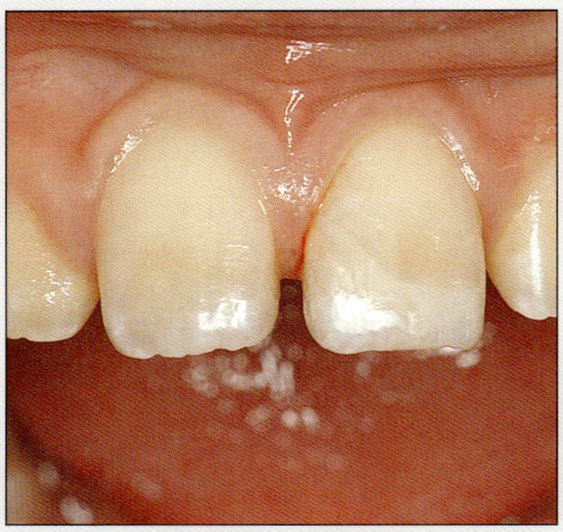

Fig 4-3j After polishing of the tooth.

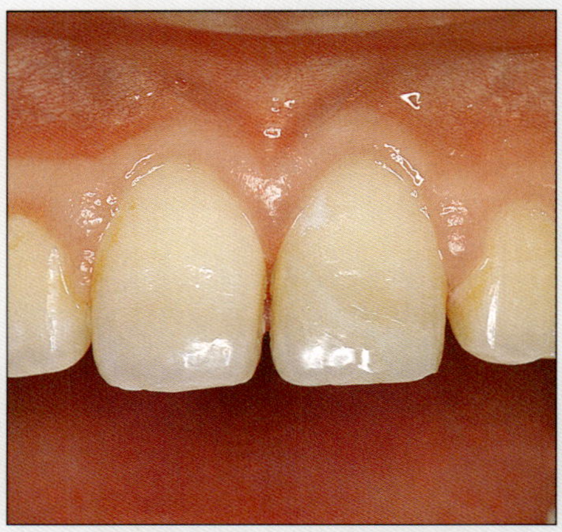

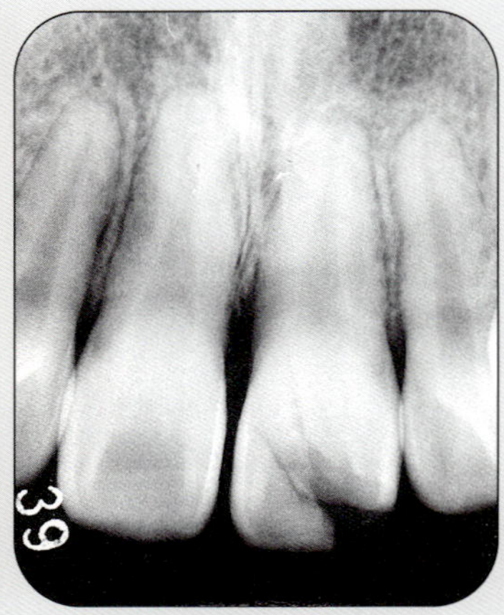

Figs 4-3k and l Five years and 3 months after treatment.

ing tooth. Fit the matrix band lightly to isolate the adhesive surface from the exudate, then apply the etchant and the bonding agent (primer) to the remaining tooth and the tooth fragment. Apply light-curing resin or chemically polymerized adhesive resin to the remaining tooth and the tooth fragment, and adapt the fractured surfaces closely. Tightening the matrix band during curing allows the tooth fragment to return to its original position buccolingually and mesiodistally (Fig 4-3i).

7. *Reshaping and polishing*: Polish with a carbide bur with a white silicone point to remove the excess composite resin and to reshape and polish the resin (Fig 4-3j).
8. *Follow-up*: Examine after 1 week, 1 month, 3 months, and 1 year. Check for discomfort, pulp necrosis, and esthetics (Figs 4-3k and l).

Fig 4-4 Treatment procedures for complicated crown-root fracture

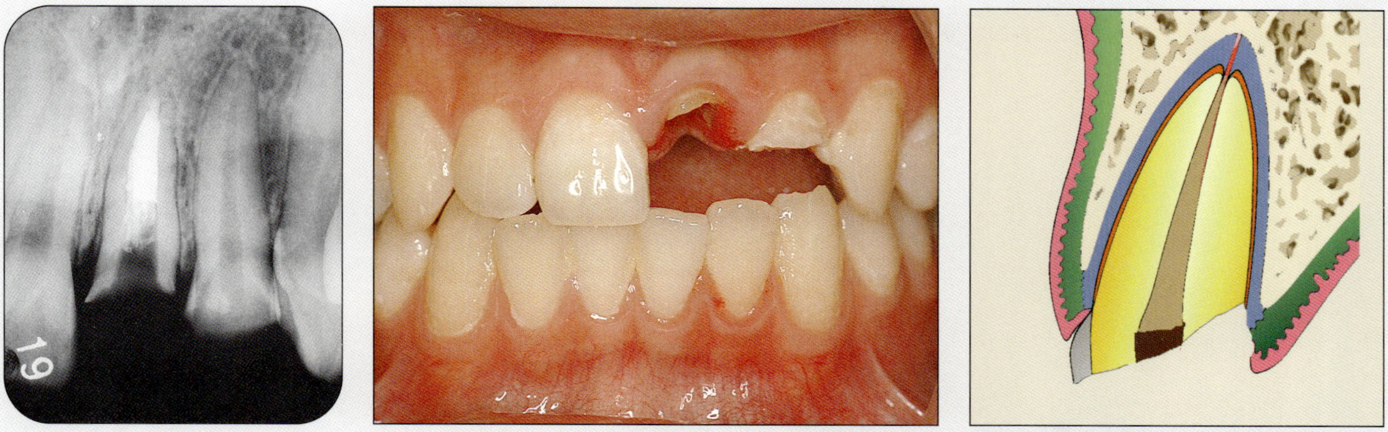

Fig 4-4a to c Sixteen-year-old boy with crown-root fracture on tooth 9 and crown fracture on tooth 10.

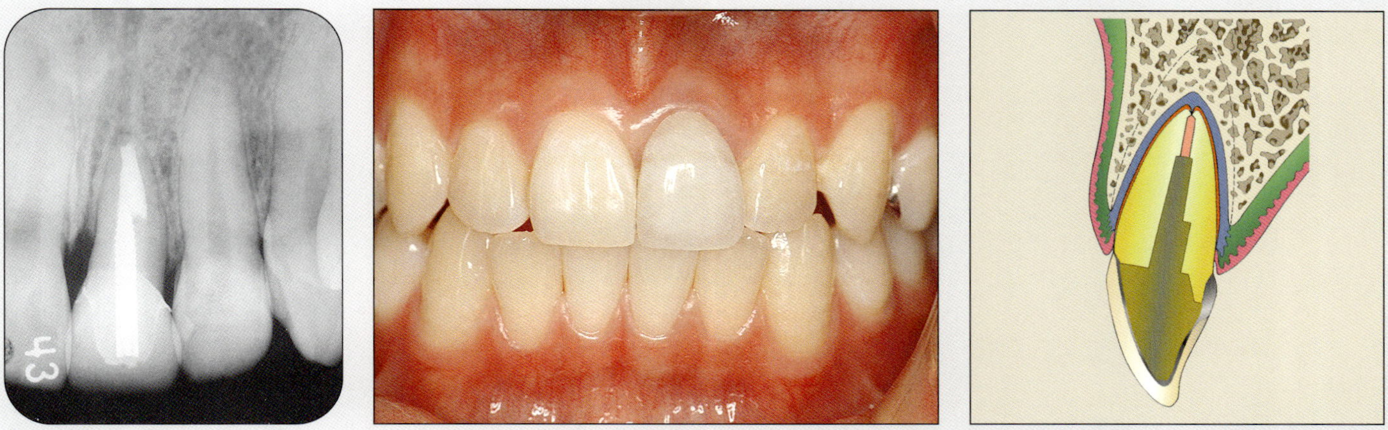

Fig 4-4d to f Postoperative views. Extrusion of root and subsequent crown restoration of tooth 9.

Complicated crown-root fracture (Fig 4-4)

If the fracture extends apical to the bony margin, it will be difficult to reattach the tooth fragment due to extensive bleeding. In some cases, the tooth fragment may not even be available. In these situations, a prosthodontic treatment approach is required. It is necessary, however, to re-establish the biologic width after extruding the root.

1. *Examination and diagnosis*: Determine whether reattachment of the tooth fragment is possible or not (Figs 4-4a and b).
2. *Removal of loose tooth fragment*: After administering anesthetic, remove the tooth fragment, if present.
3. *Root canal treatment*: For a vital tooth, use a calcium hydroxide preparation for the initial root canal filling after extirpation.
4. *Re-establishing the biologic width*: Surgically extrude the root to keep at least 4 mm of sound tooth structure coronal to the bone margin. Usually, it is best to position the root surface with the deepest extent of fracture toward the labial aspect (Figs 4-4g to l).

Fig 4-4 (Continued)

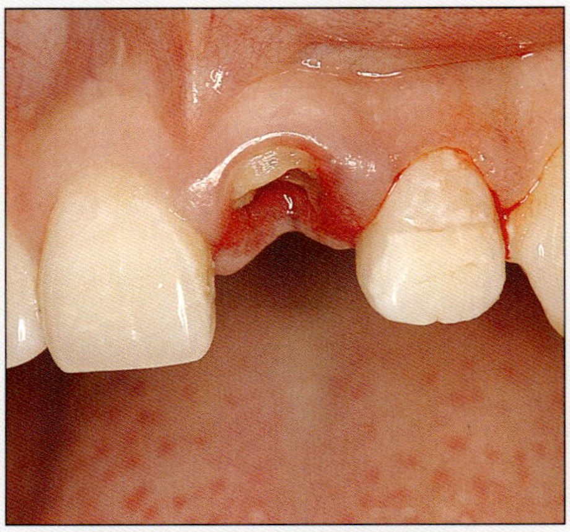

Fig 4-4g Preoperative view, after reattachment of the tooth fragment on tooth 10.

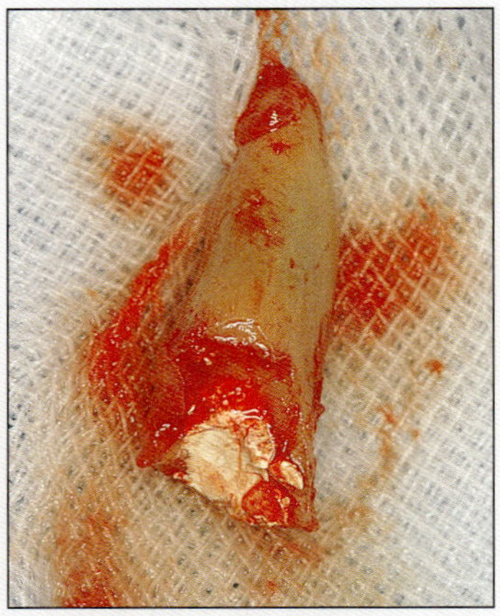

Fig 4-4h Temporary extraction of the remaining root (determine whether or not there is additional root fracture).

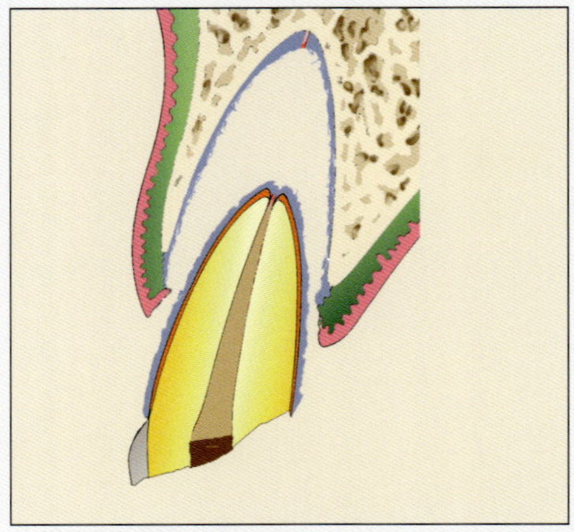

Fig 4-4i Note that half of the periodontal membrane is attached to the root.

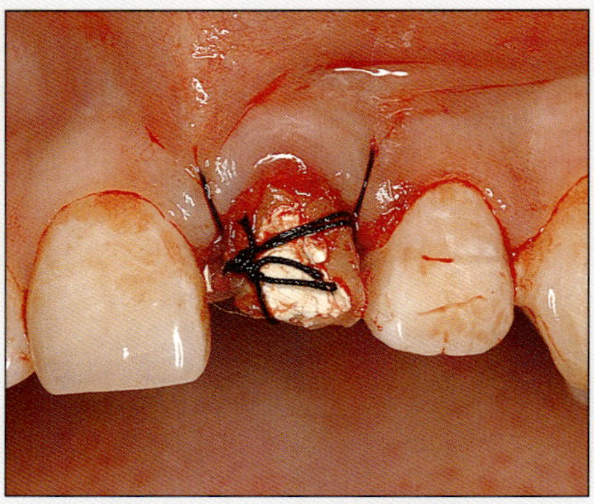

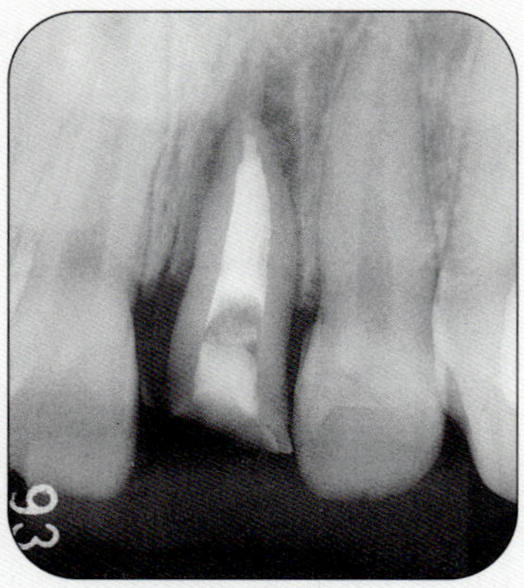

Fig 4-4j The root is rotated 180 degrees (palatal aspect at the labial aspect) and replanted into the alveolus with about 4 mm of extrusion. Sutures are used for stabilization.

Fig 4-4k After surgical extrusion.

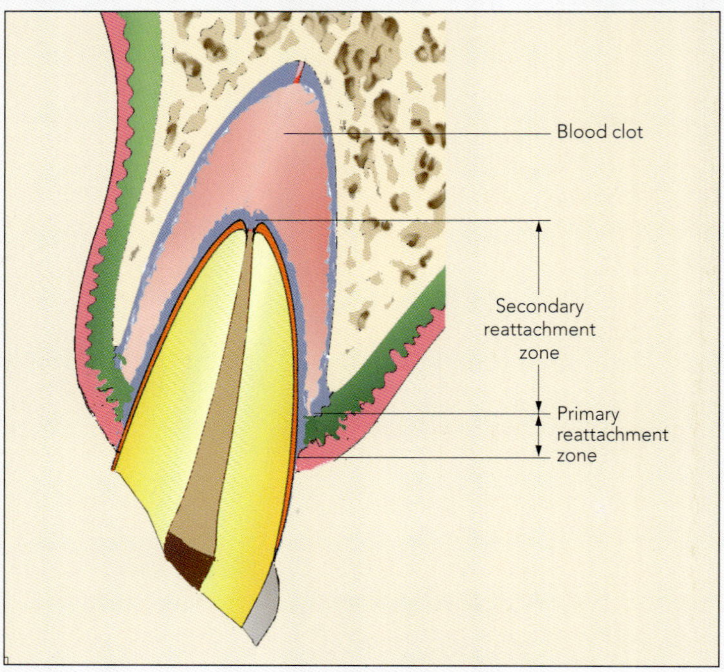

Fig 4-4l The healing mechanism after surgical extrusion.

Primary reattachment zone
2–7 days: Reattachment occurs between the periodontal membrane on the root and the gingival connective tissue.

Secondary reattachment zone
0–1 week: Blood clot occupies space between the root and alveolar cavity.
1–2 weeks: Blood clot is replaced by bony granulation tissue.
4–8 weeks: Bony granulation tissue is replaced by bone.

Fig 4-4 (Continued)

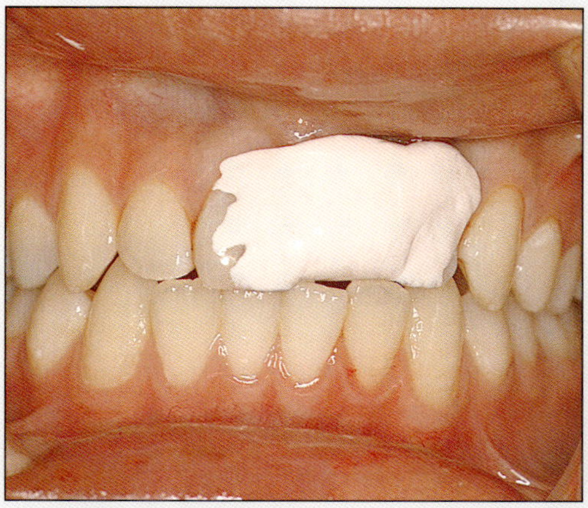

Fig 4-4m Surgical dressing is placed after surgery.

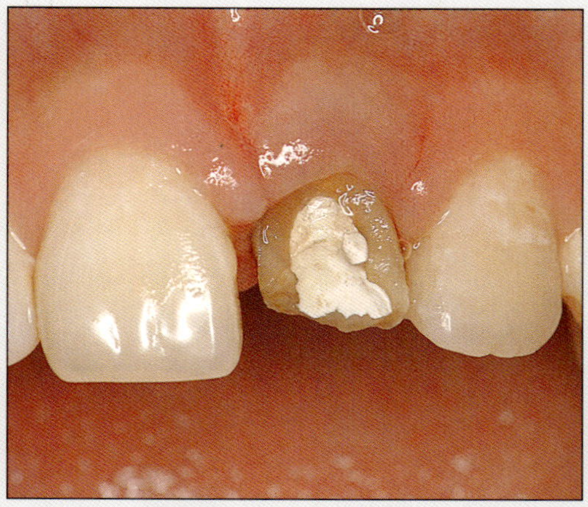

Fig 4-4n Sutures and surgical dressing are removed after 5 days.

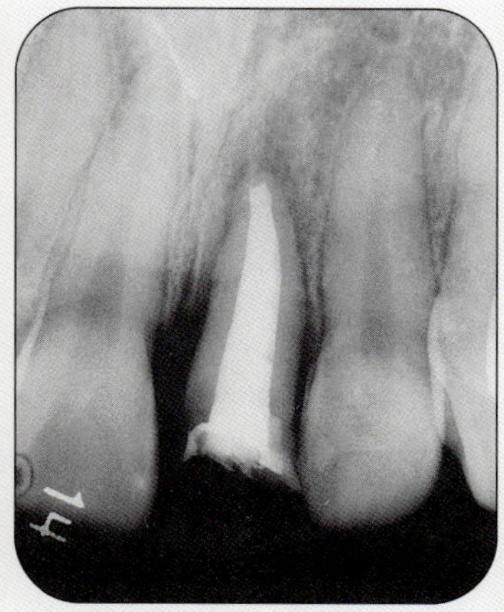

Fig 4-4o Follow-up radiograph 1 month postoperatively.

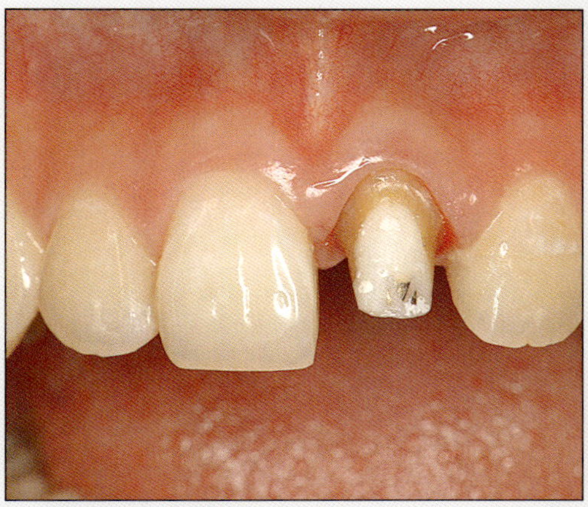

Fig 4-4p Resin core build-up.

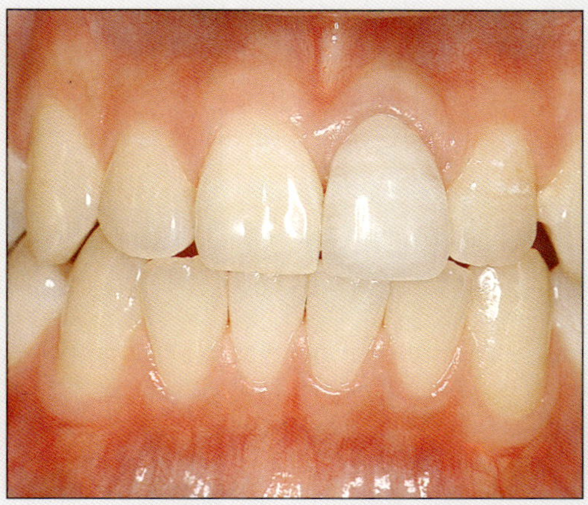

Fig 4-4q After placement of the all-ceramic restoration.

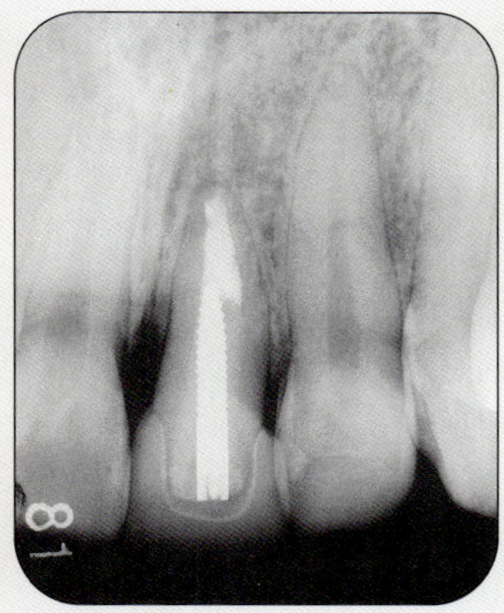

Fig 4-4r Follow-up radiograph 2 years postoperatively.

5. *Confirmation of healing*: Monitor progress until the wound has healed completely (Figs 4-4m to o).
6. *Root canal filling*: When the apical area has filled, replace the calcium hydroxide preparation with sealer and gutta-percha points (Fig 4-4o).
7. *Crown restoration*: Teeth with this type of injury usually require a post and core for prosthetic support (Figs 4-4p and q). Crown restoration with composite resin, however, is possible if sufficient sound tooth structure remains.
8. *Follow-up*: Check for root resorption or pocket formation (Fig 4-4r).

Fig 4-5 Significance of re-establishing biologic width

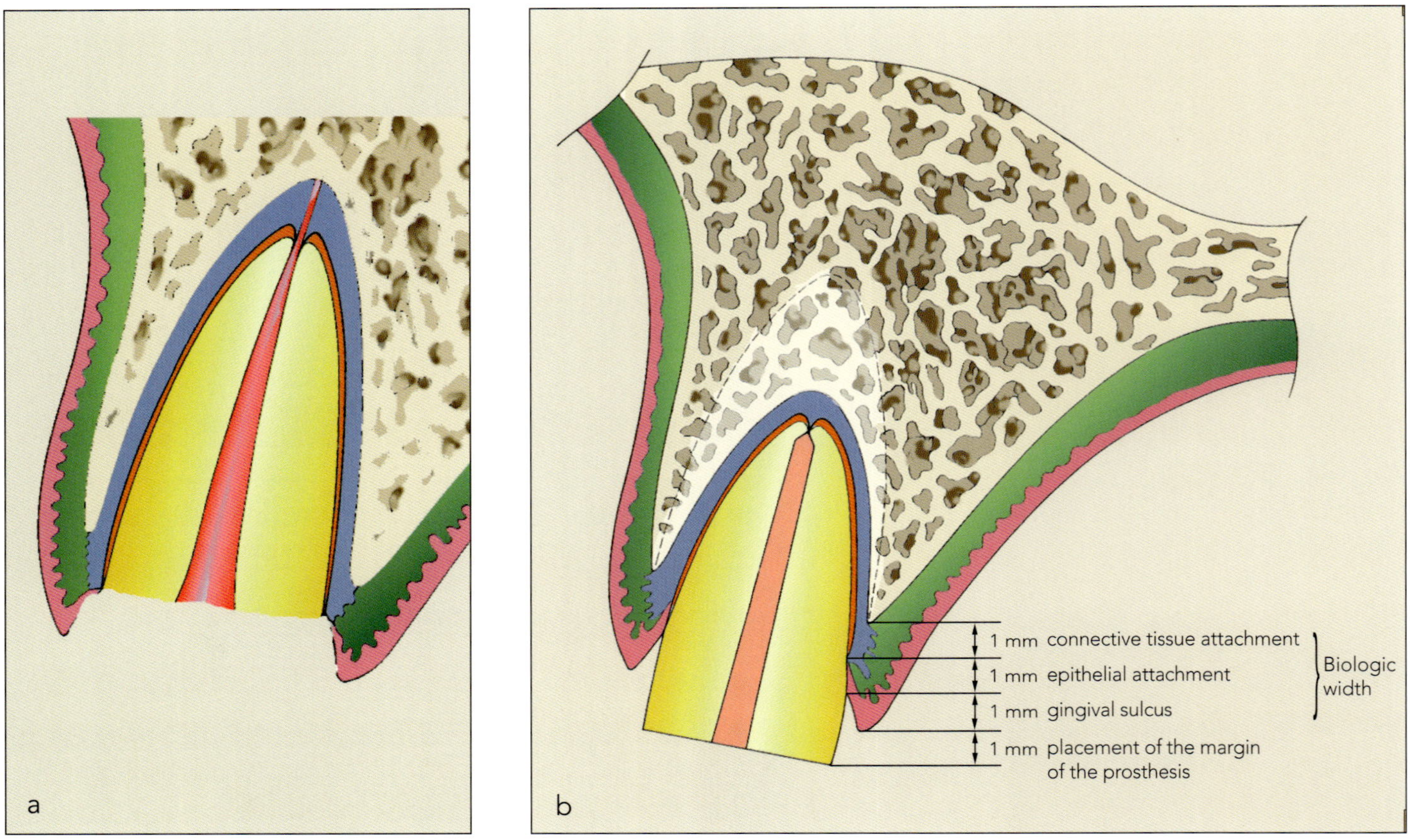

Figs 4-5a and b To re-establish biologic width, at least 4 mm of sound tooth structure should be preserved coronal to the alveolar bone margin. It is important to have about 1 mm of gingival sulcus and about 1 mm of tooth structure for the placement of the margin of the prosthesis in addition to 2 mm of the original biologic width (about 1 mm connective tissue attachment and about 1 mm epithelial attachment). (a) Preoperatively. Biologic width is lost. (b) After re-establishment of biologic width.

Re-establishing Biologic Width

Significance

Biologic width is about 2 mm. This includes about 1 mm of connective tissue attachment coronal to the bony margin and about 1 mm of epithelial attachment. Alternatively, it may be about 3 mm in width, with 1 mm of connective tissue attachment, 1 mm of epithelial attachment, and about 1 mm of healthy gingival sulcus (Fig 4-5).[24-27] Two to 3 mm of biologic width should exist on all teeth to protect the body from progression of infection from the gingival sulcus into the periodontium. Therefore, it is important not to destroy or invade the biologic width during restorative procedures. If the biologic width is lost, it must be re-established before restorative treatment.[25-27]

For biologic width, there should be about 3 mm of tooth structure coronal to the bony margin. However, it is often wise to add another 1 mm of tooth structure because the margin of the prosthesis should be placed on sound tooth structure near the gingival margin.

Fig 4-6 Treatment procedures for orthodontic extrusion

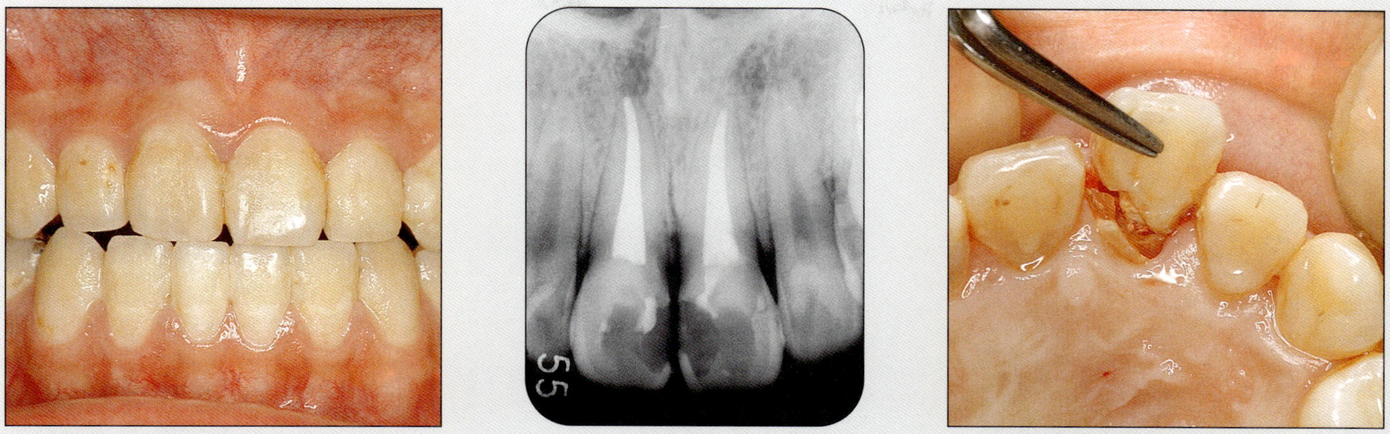

Figs 4-6a to c Preoperative views. Fourteen-year-old girl with crown-root fracture of a tooth that had undergone endodontic treatment.

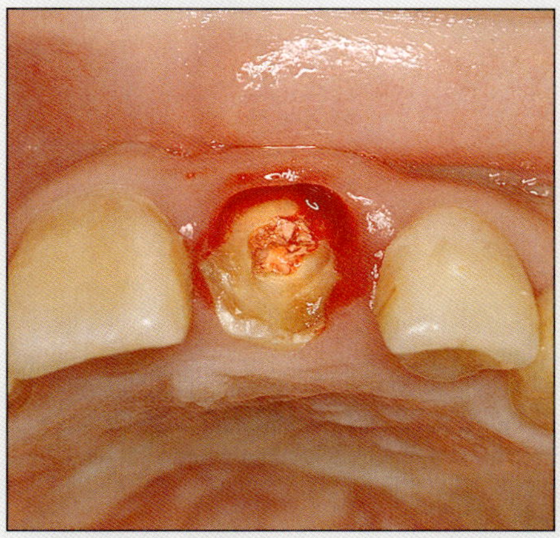

Fig 4-6d Removal of the tooth fragment.

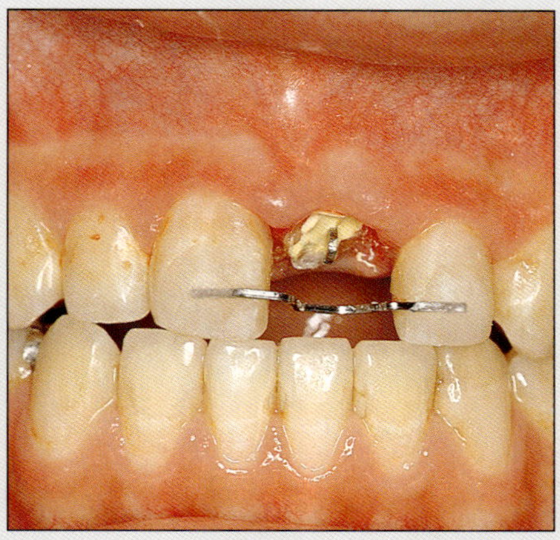

Fig 4-6e Appliance for orthodontic extrusion using an elastic band.

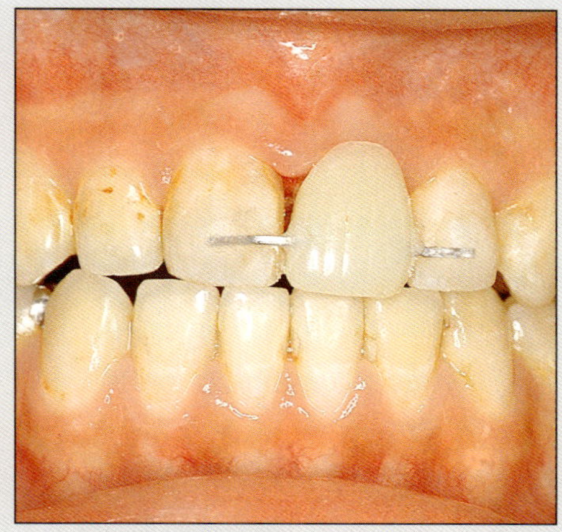

Fig 4-6f Placement of a resin shell for esthetic purposes during the procedure. The cervical line should be 1 to 2 mm from the gingival margin not to interfere with extrusion.

Methods

Methods for re-establishing biologic width lost due to caries or trauma are orthodontic extrusion, surgical extrusion, and the use of the apically positioned flap with osseous surgery.

Orthodontic extrusion. Extrude the root to provide about 4 mm of sound tooth structure coronal to the bony margin by minor tooth movement[28–30] (Figs 4-6a to f). Biologic width cannot be established by orthodontic extrusion alone because the gingiva or the alveolar bone moves coronally following tooth movement by orthodontic extrusion. Additionally, the gingival cervical line moves coronally following extrusion, causing esthetic problems (Fig 4-6g). Therefore, periodontal surgery is required after orthodontic extrusion to reshape the gingiva and the alveolar bone (Fig 4-6i). (The author performs periodontal surgery immediately after the completion of extrusion.) Avoidance of relapse after orthodontic extrusion is achieved by inserting the scalpel into the periodontal membrane, parallel to the root surface, and cutting the annular ligaments. Prosthodontic treatment is begun 2 to 3 months after surgery (Figs 4-6j to l).

Fig 4-6 (Continued)

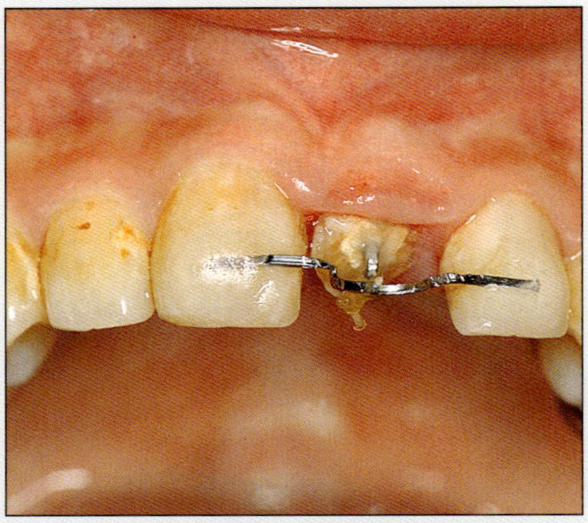

Fig 4-6g After extrusion. The gingiva has moved coronally, causing esthetic problems.

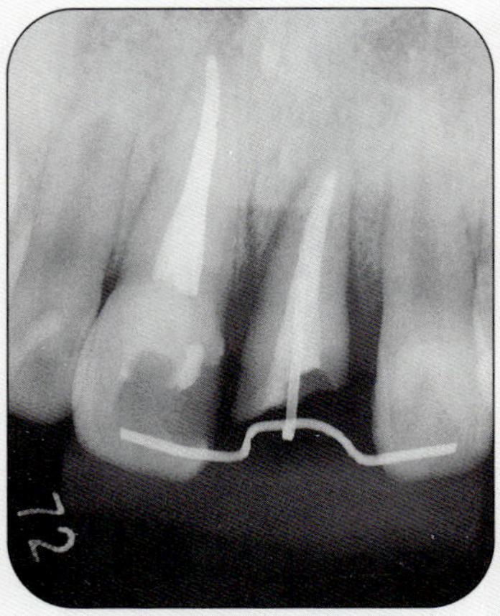

Fig 4-6h After extrusion.

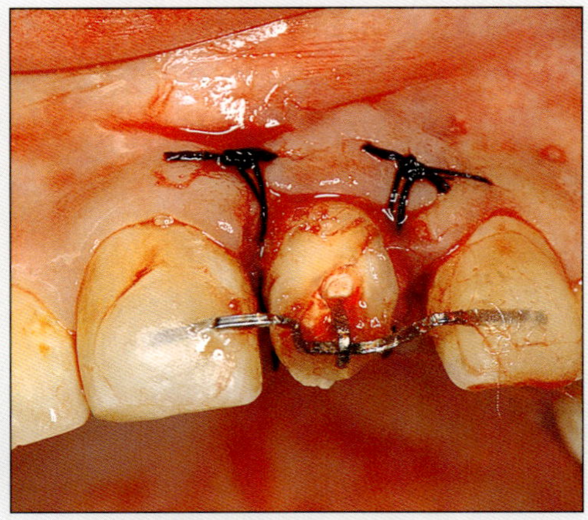

Fig 4-6i Apically positioned flap. The labial gingiva is moved apically with care not to destroy the interdental papilla. Osteoplasty or ostectomy may be required. Incision of the periodontal membrane may be necessary to avoid relapse after orthodontic extrusion.

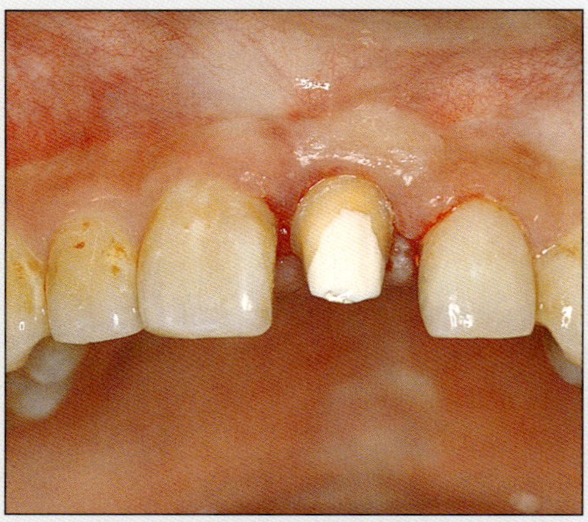

Fig 4-6j Two weeks after periodontal surgery. A provisional restoration is placed until final prosthodontic treatment is performed (2 to 3 months later).

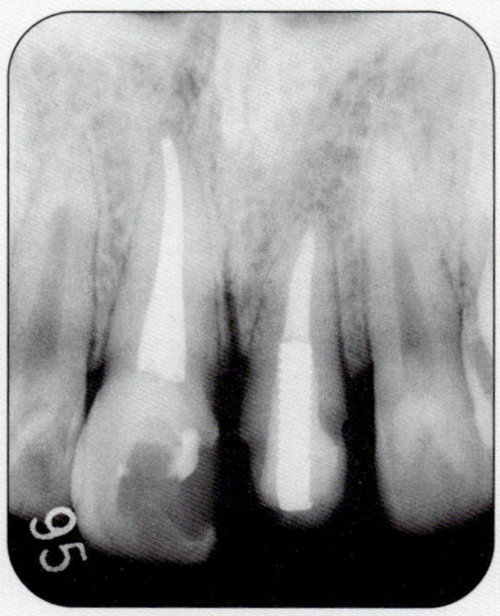

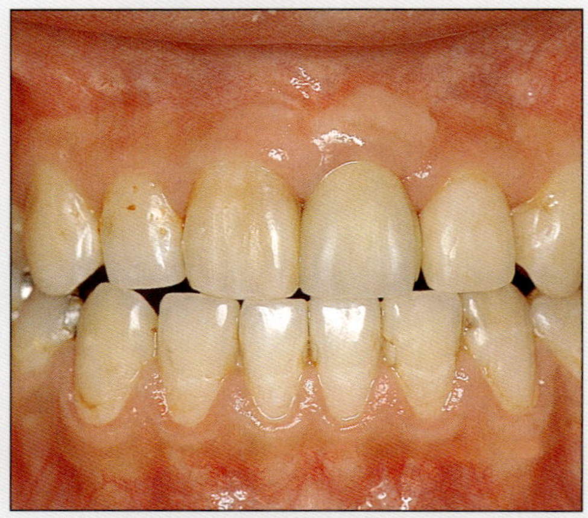

Figs 4-6k and l About 1 year and 6 months after the initial examination.

Surgical extrusion. Surgical extrusion enables repositioning of the root by placing the tooth to the desired position (including rotation) followed by stabilization (see Fig 4-4).[31,32] This procedure is called intra-alveolar transplantation. Advantages of this method are that the procedure is relatively simple and that the amount of root extrusion and movement, including rotation, can be completed as needed without relapse. The predictability is reasonably high, but failure is more frequent than with orthodontic extrusion.

The indications for surgical extrusion are limited to round-shaped roots (less divergence and concavity) and conical roots (thin toward the apex). Also, it is suitable if the deepest part of the fracture line is not on the labial aspect. Positioning the shortest part of the root labially is the principal advantage of this method. The labial bony margin of the alveolar bone is lower than it is on the palatal side. Therefore, positioning the shortest part of the root on that aspect during extrusion achieves the purpose of the extrusion while keeping as much root in the alveolar bone as possible (Figs 4-4g to k). The repair mechanism of the wound in surgical extrusion is basically reattachment. In a few days, reattachment between the gingival connective tissue and the periodontal membrane of the root surface will occur. Within 2 weeks to 2 months, reattachment will occur in the alveolus[33,34] (Fig 4-4l).

Apically positioned flap with osseous surgery. Biologic width can also be established by raising the gingival flap and exposing the root by removing the supporting bone around the root.[27,35–37] The gingival flap is placed apically to cover 1 to 2 mm of root to the same level as the gingiva.

This method has limitations, however. It may be clinically difficult to expose 3 mm of root because of the large amount of bone removal required. Also, it may not be esthetically acceptable because of the very inconsistent topography created between the adjacent teeth. This method is not applicable under such conditions.

5

Root Fracture

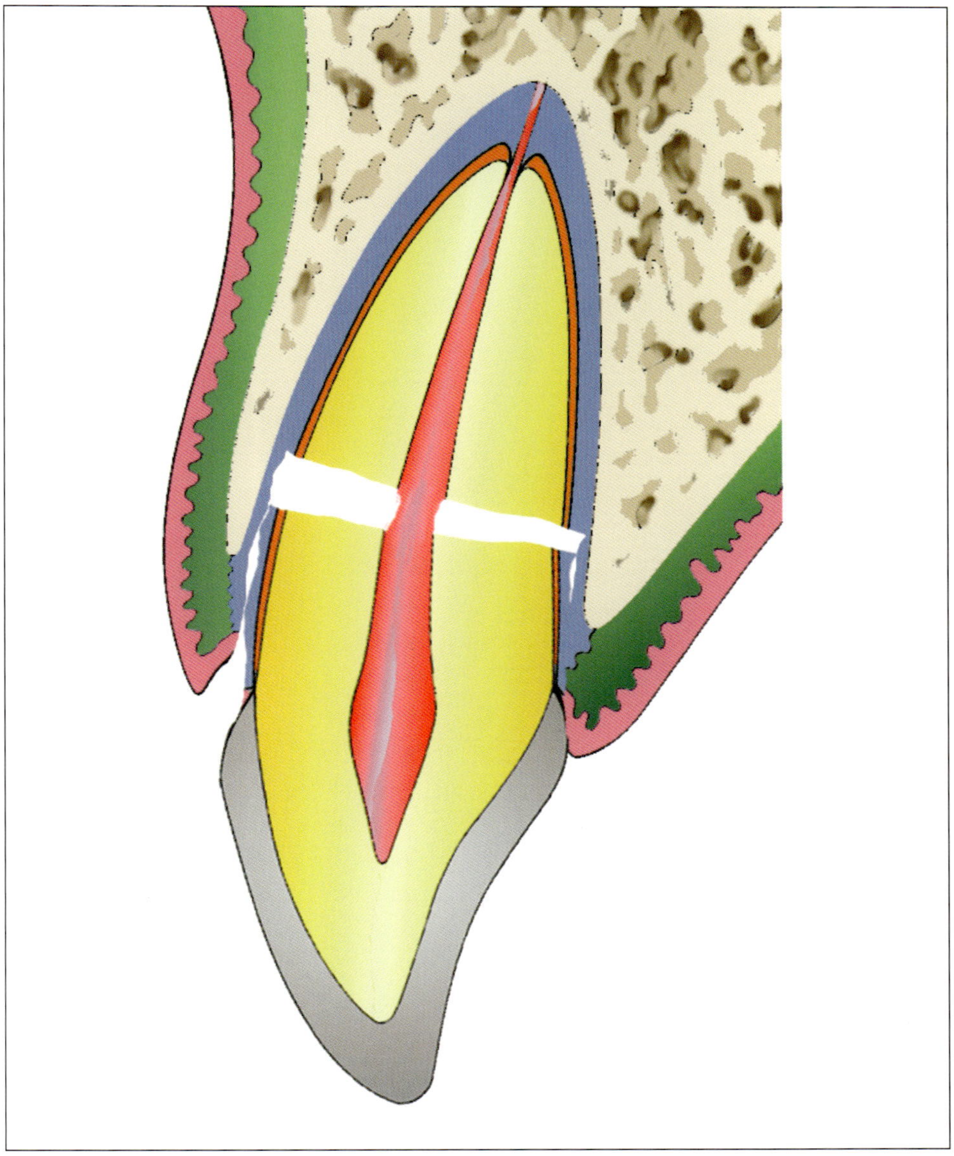

Root fractures are infrequent injuries, which may be why they are often incorrectly treated (ie, unnecessary root canal treatment). Because the coronal segment of a root-fractured tooth often is luxated and even avulsed, root fracture injuries may require treatment for such injuries in addition to management of the root fracture.

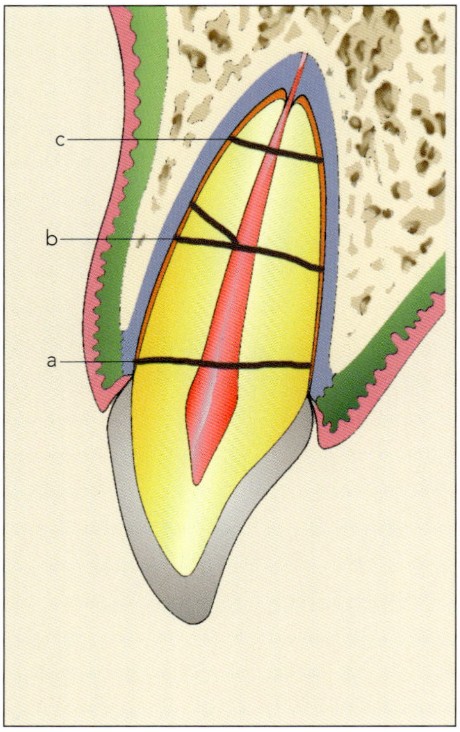

Fig 5-1 Root fractures. (a) Shallow root fracture. (b and c) Deep root fracture.

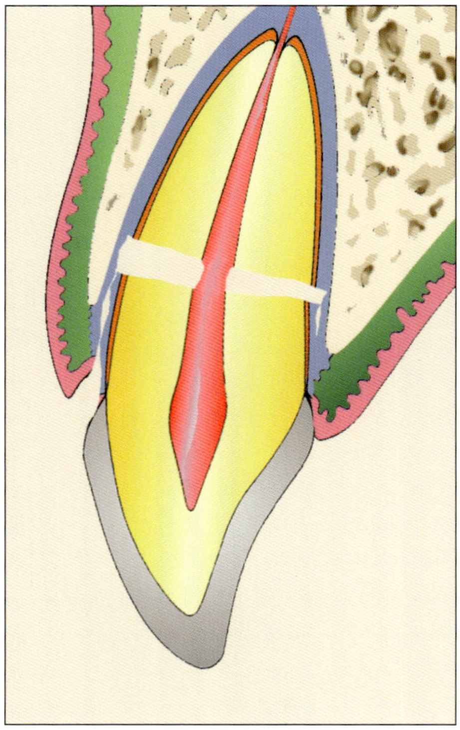

Fig 5-2 Root fracture without necrosis of the pulp.

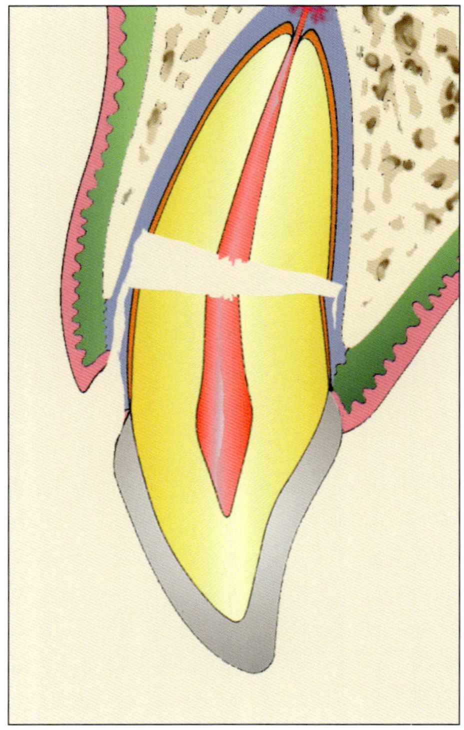

Fig 5-3 Root fracture with necrosis of the pulp. There are two types of necrosis of the pulp: that caused by severance of the pulp between the fractured segments of the root (necrosis of the pulp occurs in the coronal region only) and that caused by vascular damage in the apical area (necrosis of entire pulp).

Description

The root fracture involves the cementum, dentin, and pulp. The fracture line (or lines) may be well within the bony support, in which case it is considered a *deep root fracture* (Fig 5-1[b and c]), or the fracture line is at or close to the crestal bone of the alveolus and is called a *shallow root fracture* (Fig 5-1[a]).

Examination and Diagnosis: Key Points

Prudence is required in examining and diagnosing root fractures. Sometimes during the initial examination, obvious tooth crown malposition or fracture lines are undetected by inspection or radiography (see Chapter 2, Case 4). Also, the position and the direction of the fracture line varies mesiodistally and buccolingually, and the radiographic image is affected by the direction of the X-ray beam. Therefore, in cases without malposition of the crown, radiographs need to be taken at different angles.

The electric pulp test (EPT) should always be performed. With this test, it is possible to detect fragmentation of the pulp. Even if the radiograph suggests fragmentation of the pulp, the pulp is not necessarily severed, in which case root canal treatment can be avoided (Fig 5-2). Conversely, when response to the EPT is negative, there could be severance of the pulp at the fracture site or vascular severance of the apex due to subluxation of the apical root fragment (Fig 5-3). Additionally, vascular severance of the apex may occur without severance of the pulp at the fracture site. In such cases, there will be necrosis of the entire pulp.

Inspection and palpation provide information about the degree of tooth malposition. If there is extensive malposition and the fractured surface is exposed to the oral cavity, there is a strong possibility that there will be severance of the pulp and infection of the pulp tissue coronally. It is essential to understand the condition of the root fracture because the treatment plan varies depending on the involvement of the pulp and the position and direction of the fracture line.

Treatment Plan

Deep root fracture

Reduce the fracture by repositioning the segments, and splint the tooth to the adjacent teeth. The current recommendation is to splint for up to 3 months (Fig 5-4). When there is evidence of pulp necrosis, proceed with endodontic treatment as described below (Fig 5-5).

Shallow root fracture

If the remaining root is deemed adequate to support a prosthetic crown, the root must be extruded either surgically or orthodontically as described for crown-root fractures (see Chapter 4). A short root may be an indication for extraction. If extraction is chosen, consider the esthetic and functional recovery possibilities with autotransplantation (Fig 5-6), an implant, a fixed partial denture, or orthodontic closure of the space.

Treatment Procedures

Case with no pulp necrosis (Fig 5-4)

1. *Examination and diagnosis*: Determine the location of the root fracture by radiographic examination, and check for pulp response to the EPT (Figs 5-4a to c).
2. *Local anesthesia*: Administer local anesthetic as necessary.
3. *Repositioning and splinting*: Reposition the coronal tooth fragment to its original position as closely as possible and splint it with an adhesive resin and wire (1 × 3 twisted wire, 3M Unitek) (Figs 5-4d to f).
4. *Follow-up*: Perform clinical examination, radiographic examination, and EPT 1 week, 1 month, and 3 months after the initial treatment. Check for pulp necrosis, inflammation of the fracture site, and discomfort. Remove the splint if the pulp responds normally and the radiographic findings are favorable. (The splinting period is about 3 months.)

If the coronal segment remains very mobile after splint removal, it may be necessary to continue the re-splint for a longer period of time (Figs 5-4g to i).

Fig 5-4 Treatment plan for deep root fracture without pulp necrosis

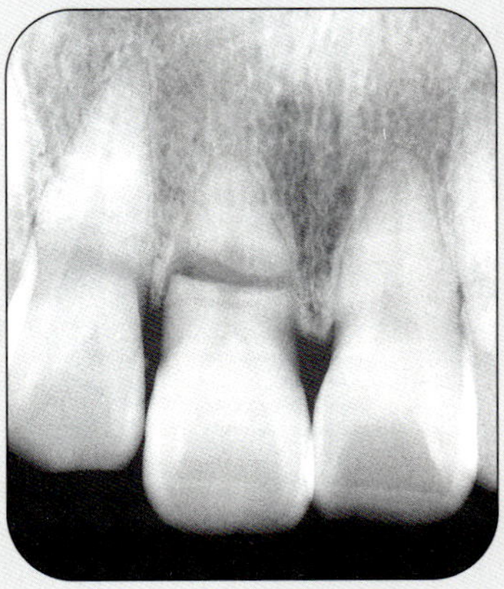
Fig 5-4a

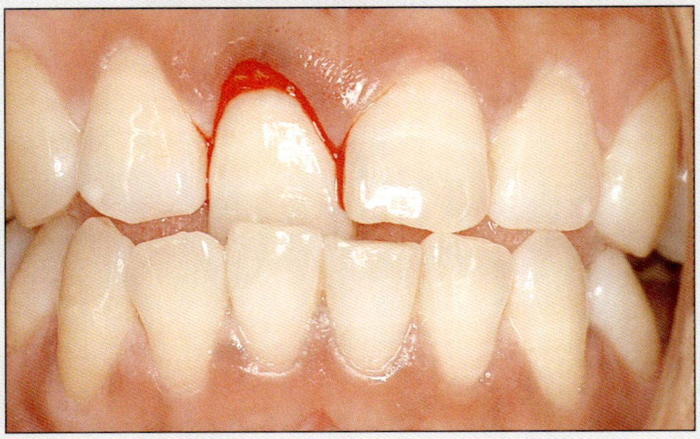
Fig 5-4b

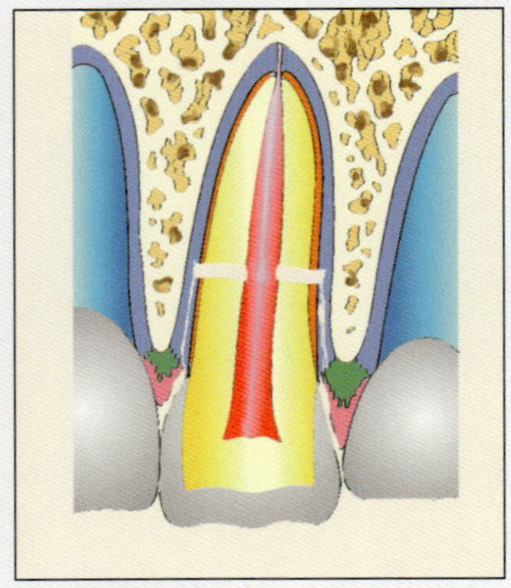
Fig 5-4c

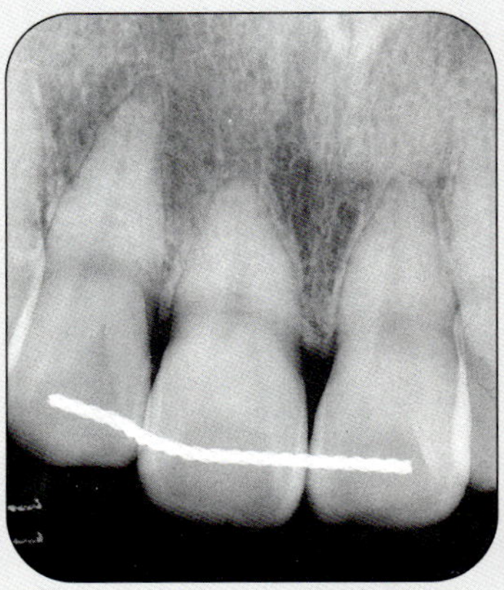
Fig 5-4d

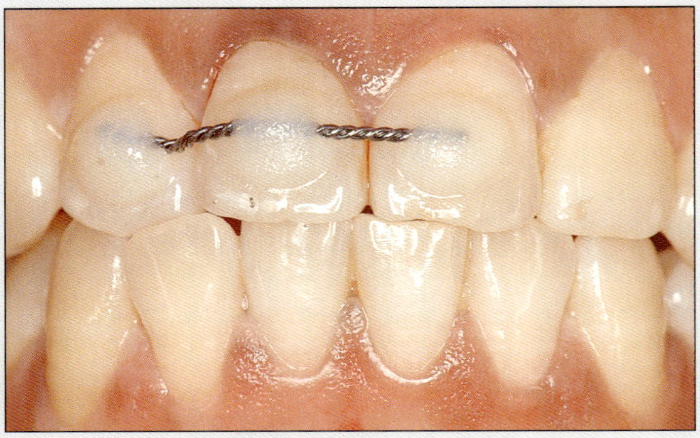
Fig 5-4e

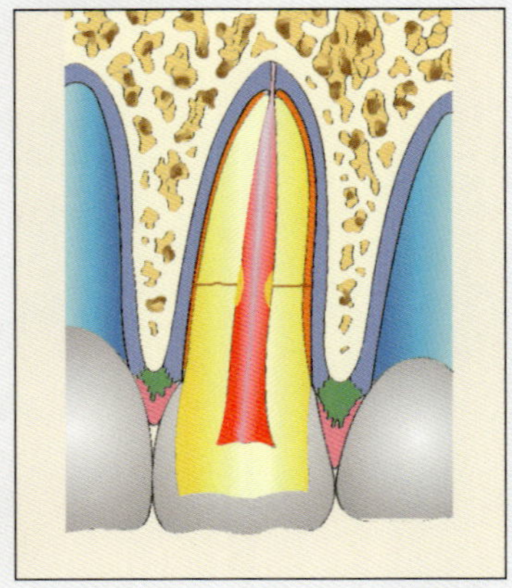
Fig 5-4f

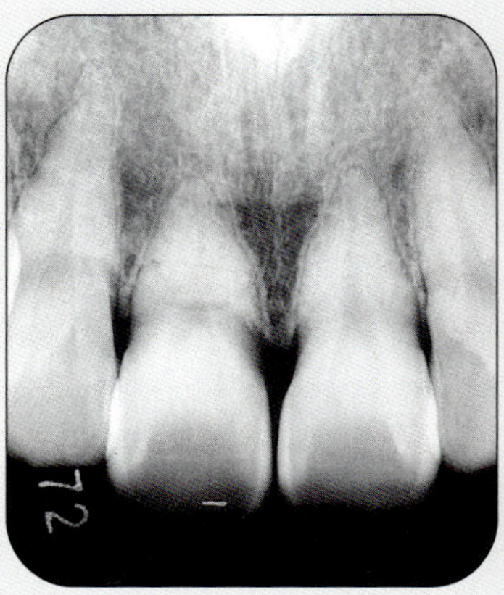
Fig 5-4g

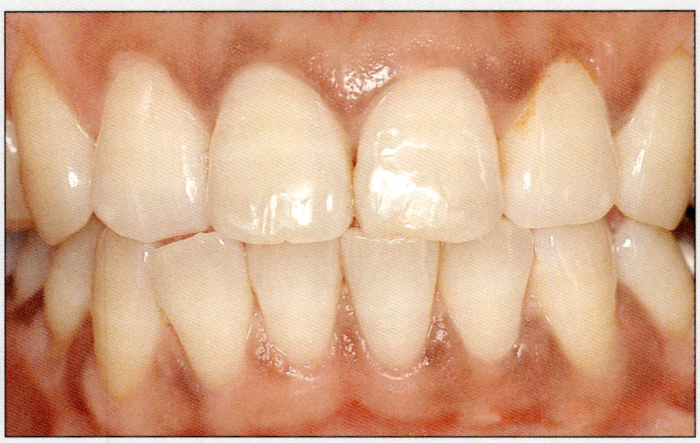
Fig 5-4h

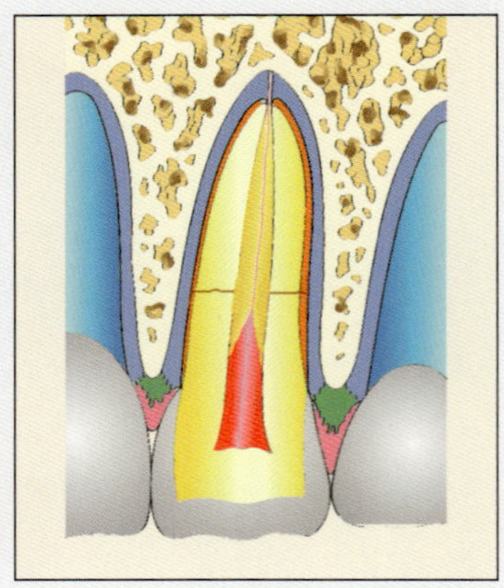
Fig 5-4i

Figs 5-4a to c Preoperative views, 31-year-old woman. The pulp is vital.

Figs 5-4d and e After repositioning and splinting.

Fig 5-4f Ideal healing after reduction of fracture and splinting: apposition of dentin on the pulp side of the fractured surface and apposition of cementum on the root surface.

Figs 5-4g and h Six years after treatment.

Fig 5-4i Healing. Coronal and apical fragments are joined with hard tissue (dentin and cementum) and the pulp cavity is greatly reduced.

Case with pulp necrosis (Fig 5-5)

Even if pulp vitality is unclear at the time of the initial diagnosis, it is best to treat as if the pulp is vital until and if pulp necrosis can be definitively diagnosed. However, if the negative pulp response continues, clinical discomfort such as percussion pain develops, and there is radiolucency at the fracture site, pulp necrosis exists. In such cases, follow steps 1 through 3 before removing the splint.

1. Proceed with endodontic therapy of the coronal segment to the level of the fracture only. Prepare that portion of the canal and fill it with a calcium hydroxide preparation to the level of the fracture (Figs 5-5a to f). Placement of calcium hydroxide in the coronal root canal will stimulate hard tissue formation, closing off the root canal opening from the coronal segment into the fracture space. The pulp of the apical segment will undergo hard tissue deposition, reducing the pulp canal lumen significantly (Figs 5-5g to i). After confirmation of closure, use sealer and gutta-percha or a conventional glass-ionomer cement to fill the coronal pulp cavity. The crown can be bleached if discolored, and a composite resin used for restoration. Usually with traumatized teeth, root canal obliteration occurs in the apical pulp cavity and no treatment is necessary.
2. On rare occasions, the entire pulp becomes inflamed and possibly necrotic in a tooth with root fracture. This can be recognized by continued discomfort even after coronal pulpotomy, or by the development of a lesion at the fracture site and the root apex (Figs 5-7a to c). In such cases, endodontic therapy should include both the coronal and the apical portions of the tooth. After canal preparation, place calcium hydroxide in the entire canal and wait for evidence of healing before filling the canal with gutta-percha and sealer.
3. If the root canal treatment fails in the apical segment, remove the apical fragment surgically (Figs 5-7d and e). There are two methods of accomplishing this: One is apicoectomy and the other is intentional replantation. The latter is performed by extracting the coronal tooth fragment, removing the apical tooth fragment from the socket, and replacing the coronal tooth segment to its original position. Follow Step 1 for pulp treatment of the coronal segment.

Responses to Root Fractures

There are four responses to root fracture: healing with calcified tissue, healing with interposition of fibrous connective tissue, healing with interposition of bone, and lack of healing as demonstrated by the interposition of granulation tissue[5,7] (Fig 5-8).

Healing with calcified tissue (Fig 5-8a)

If the coronal tooth segment is repositioned and splinted to its original position without irreversible pulpal injury, there will be healing with calcified tissue in the fractured root region[7] (ie, the apposition of dentin inside the pulp cavity and the apposition of cementum outside the root) (see Fig 5-4). Consequently, the root and the tooth segments will be connected by calcified tissue. Gradually, the pulp tissue, especially in the apical region, will undergo calcification (the apposition of dentin) and the pulp cavity will be obliterated.

Healing with interposition of connective tissue (Fig 5-8b)

If the coronal and apical root segments cannot be repositioned properly, interposition of blood clots in the fracture site occurs. Granulation tissue derived from pulp tissue or periodontal membrane tissue then invades and proliferates into the blood clots (Figs 5-9a and b). This granulation tissue causes areas of root resorption, pre-

Fig 5-5 Treatment plan for deep root fracture with pulp necrosis

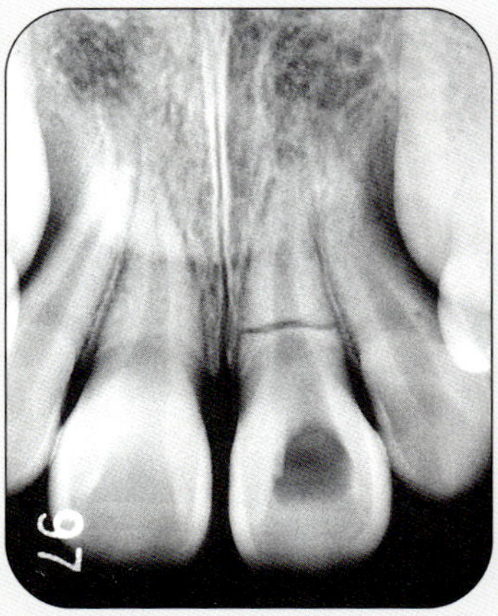
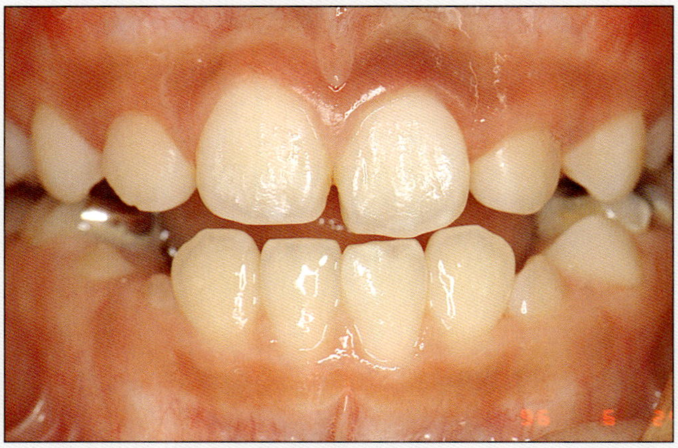

Figs 5-5a and b Preoperative views, 10-year-old girl. Pulpotomy of the coronal pulp had been performed before the current examination.

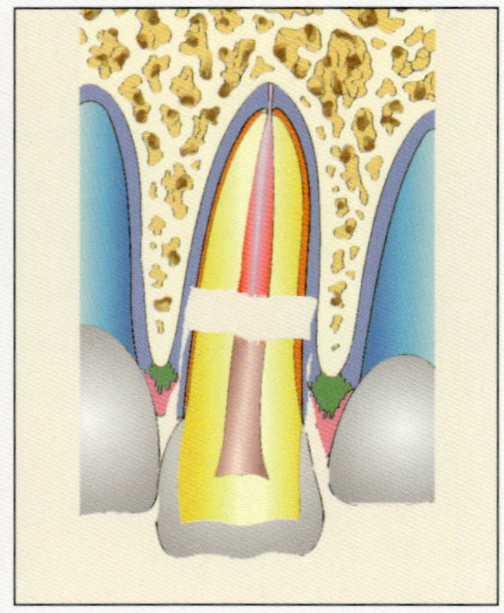

Fig 5-5c Partial (coronal) necrosis.

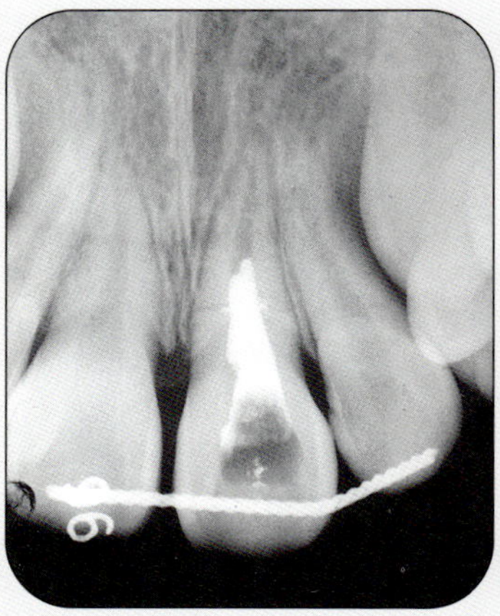
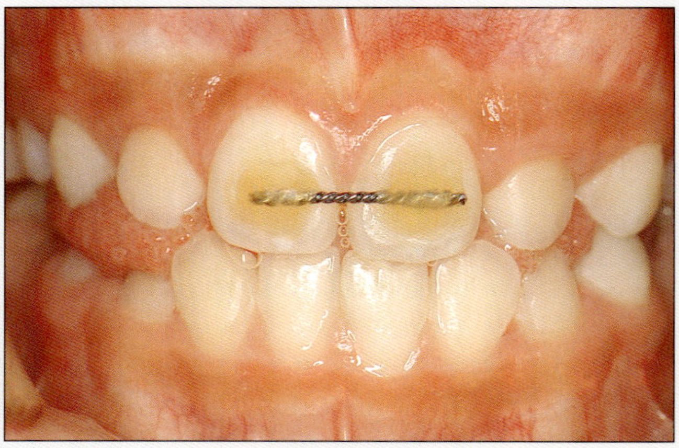

Figs 5-5d and e After repositioning, splinting, and initial endodontic treatment. The coronal part of the root canal is cleaned to where the pulp is bleeding or response to touch indicates vitality. It is then filled with a calcium hydroxide preparation.

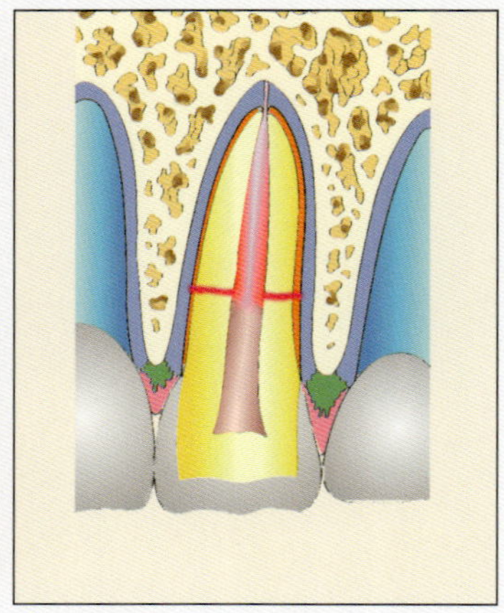

Fig 5-5f Temporary inflammation in the area of root severance.

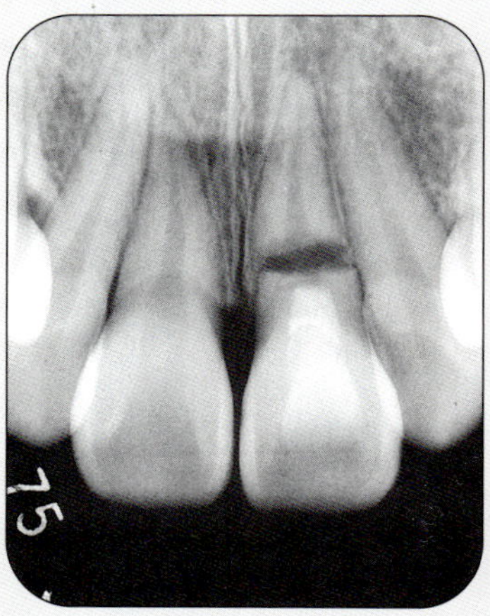
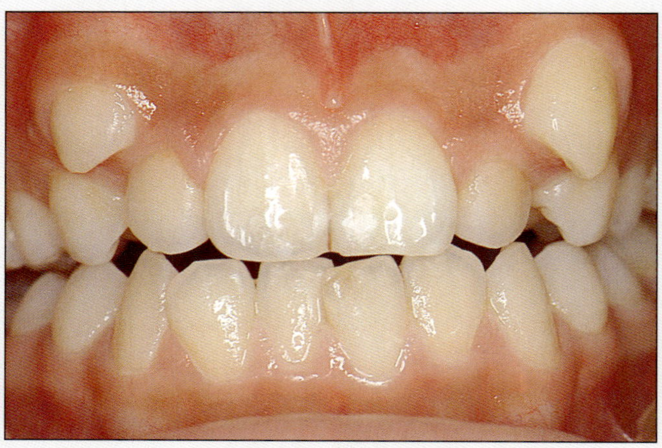

Figs 5-5g and h After restorative treatment, 1 year and 8 months after initial treatment. The calcium hydroxide preparation in the root canal was absorbed and replaced with vital tissue. The fractured surface of the coronal tooth fragment was closed with hard tissue. Because the patient was still growing, there was separation of the fractured segments. Bony tissue had invaded the separated space (Fig 5-8c).

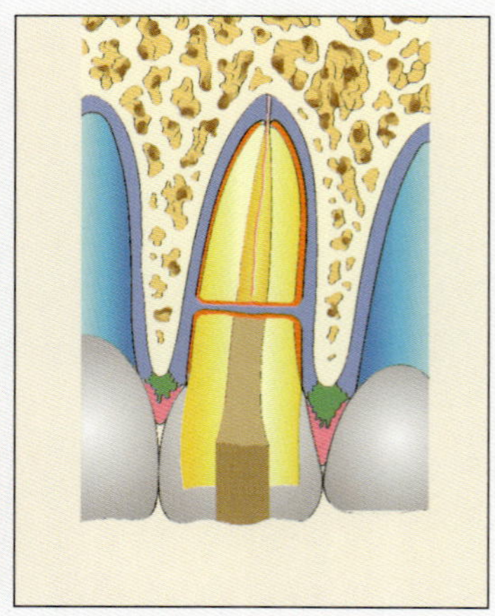

Fig 5-5i When only the coronal tooth fragment has necrotic pulp tissue, only the coronal segment requires endodontic treatment.

Fig 5-6 Autotransplantation for shallow root fracture

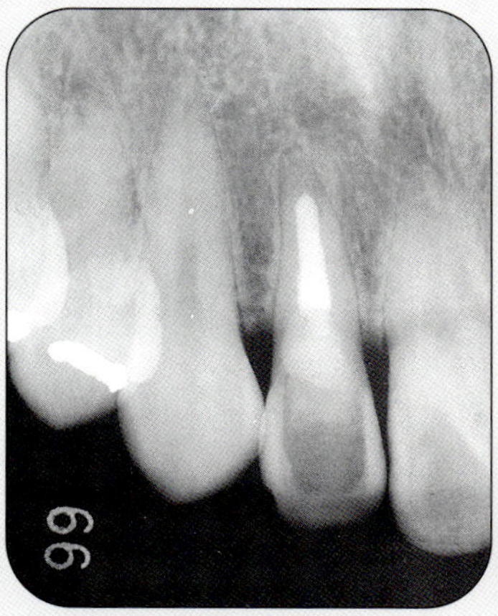

Fig 5-6a Preoperative radiograph, 34-year-old woman.

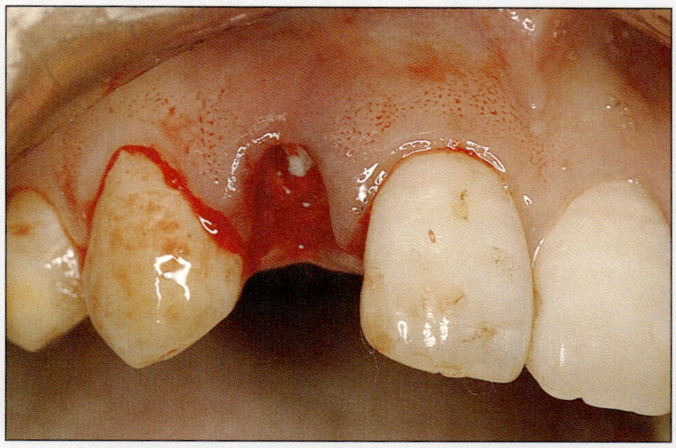

Fig 5-6b Removal of tooth fragment. The remaining short root of tooth 7 makes it difficult to extrude it for restoration.

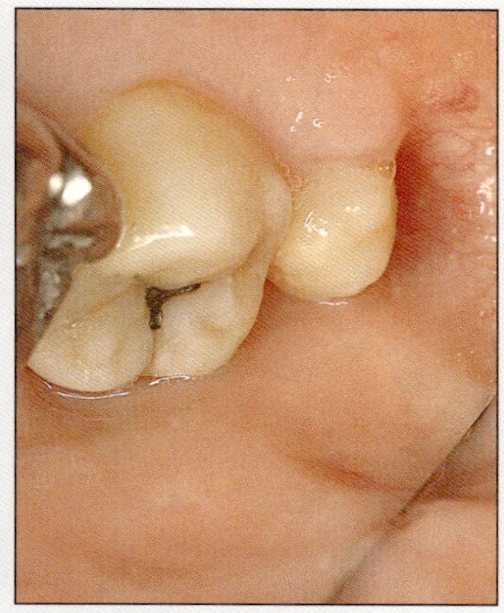

Fig 5-6c Tooth 16, a very small third molar, has been preserved.

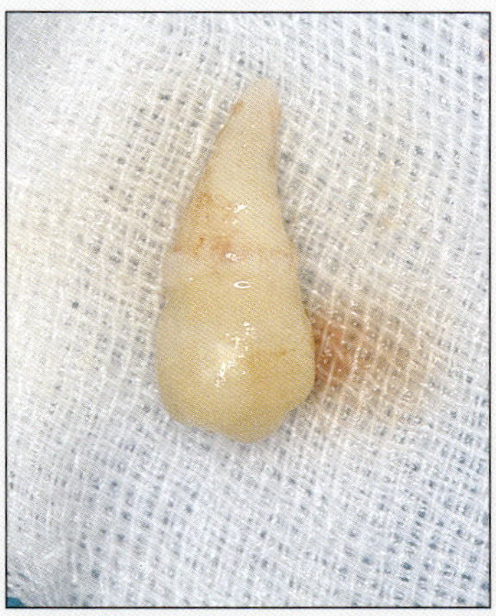

Fig 5-6d Tooth 16 is extracted for transplantation.

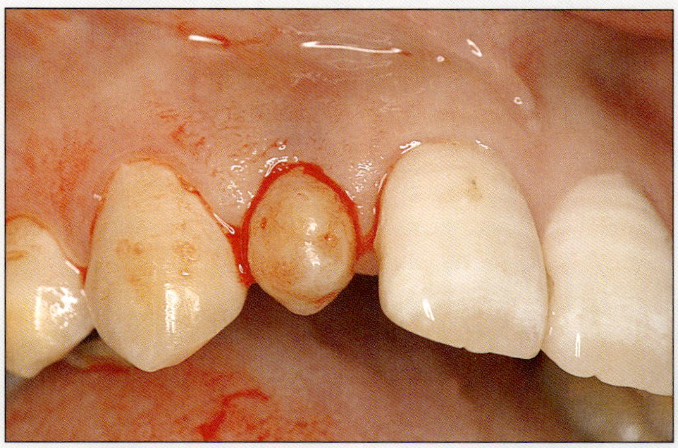

Fig 5-6e Autotransplantation: Tooth 16 is transferred to the extraction socket of tooth 7.

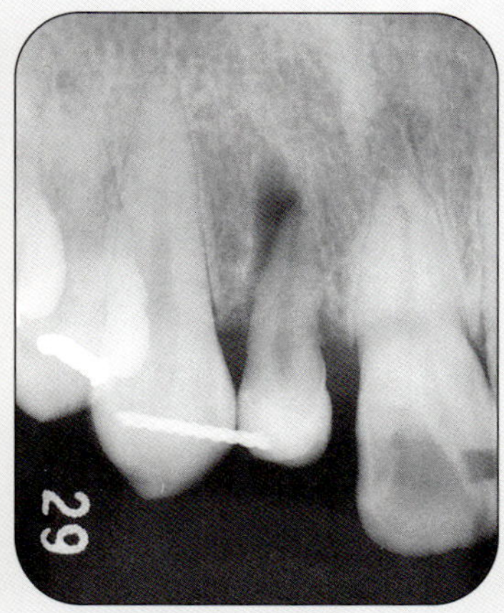

Fig 5-6f After transplantation.

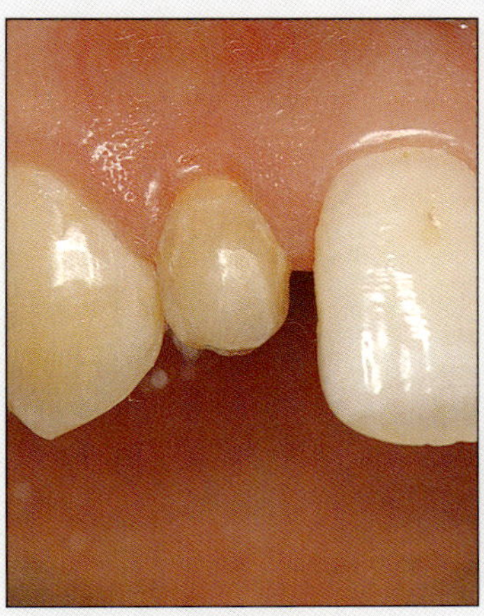

Fig 5-6g Three months after surgery.

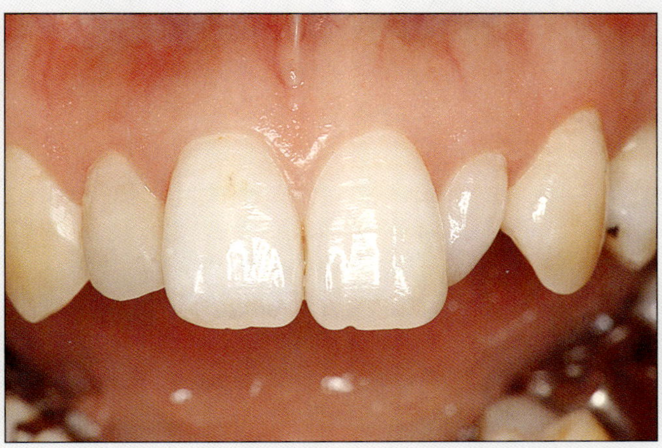

Fig 5-6h After bleaching and restorative treatment with composite resin of the transplanted tooth.

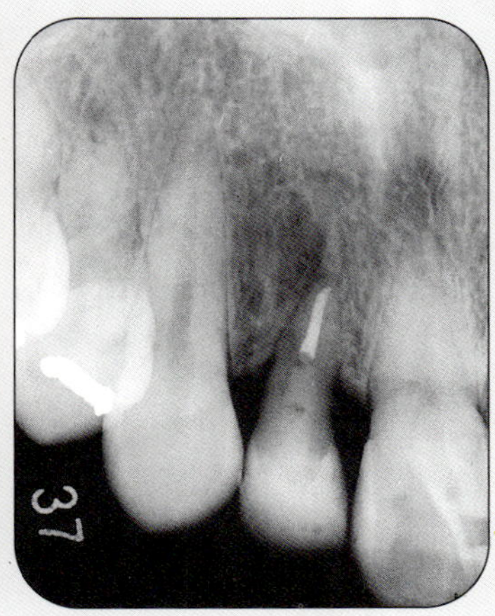

Fig 5-6i Approximately 2 years after the surgery.

Fig 5-7 Treatment plan for deep root fractures with pulp necrosis of the coronal and apical segments

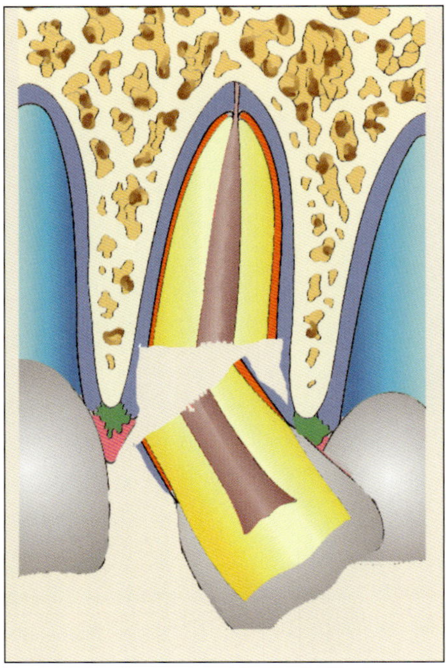

Fig 5-7a Pulp necrosis in both root segments.

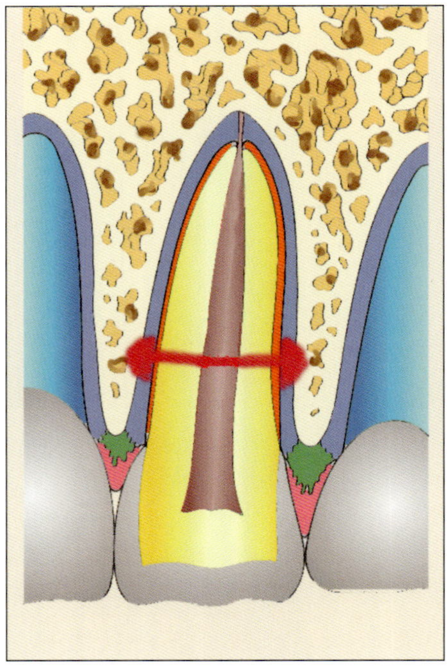

Fig 5-7b After repositioning and splinting. If pulp necrosis is left untreated, granulation tissue will develop between the root segments.

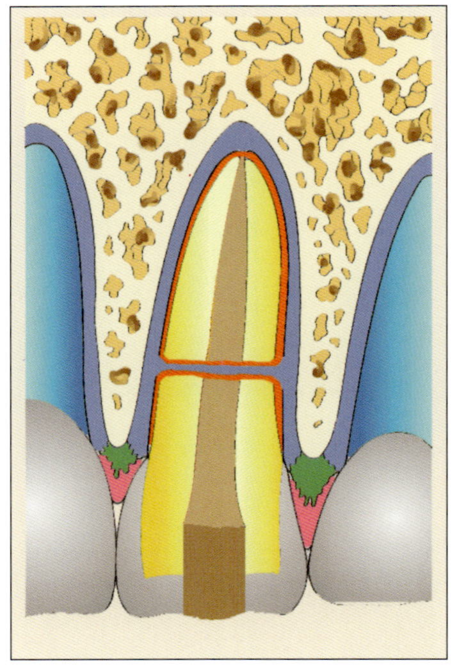

Fig 5-7c After cleansing and preparation of the entire canal, the canal is filled with a calcium hydroxide preparation.

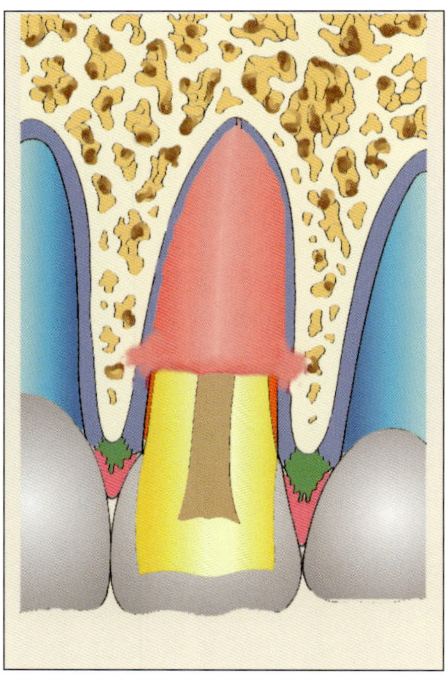

Fig 5-7d If endodontic treatment of the apical segment fails, that segment only should be removed.

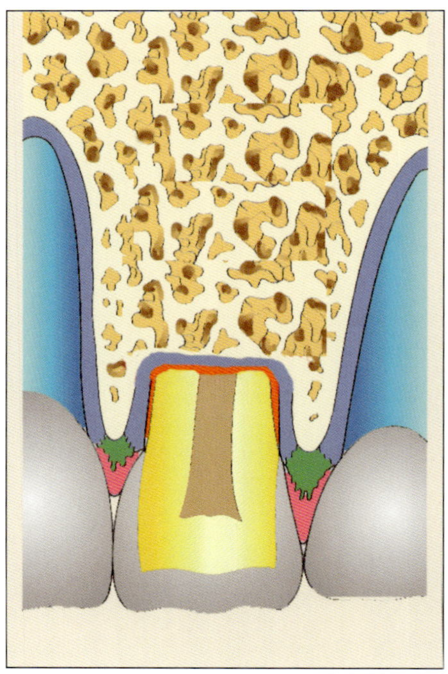

Fig 5-7e Healing. Filling the pulp cavity of the coronal segment with a calcium hydroxide preparation allows the root canal opening at the fracture site to close with cementum.

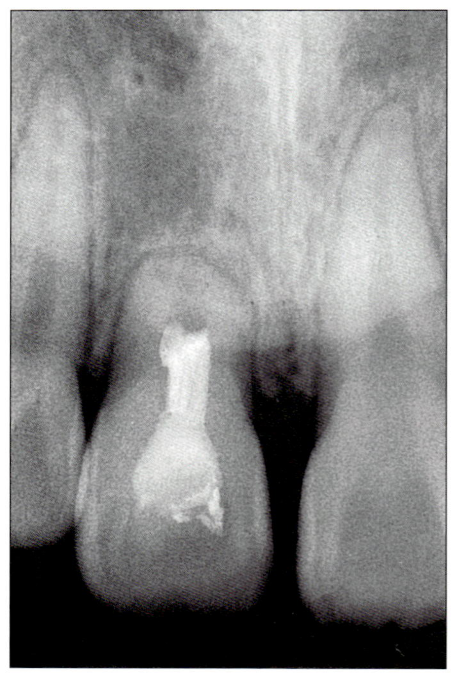

Fig 5-7f Radiograph corresponding to Fig 5-7e. (Courtesy of Dr Takayuki Sato.)

Fig 5-8 Response to repositioning and fixation of root-fractured teeth

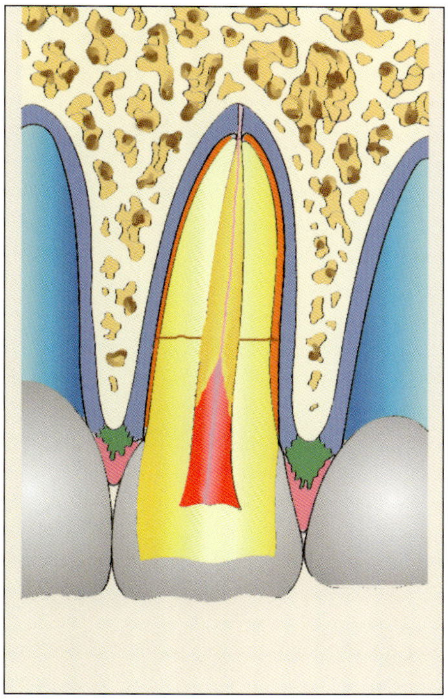

Fig 5-8a Healing with calcified tissue.

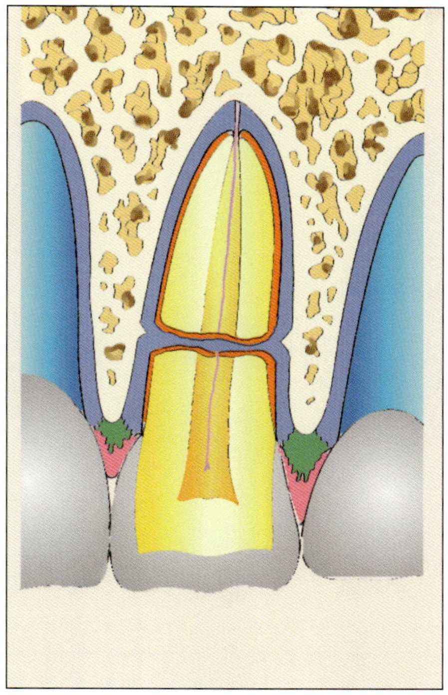

Fig 5-8b Healing with interposition of connective tissue.

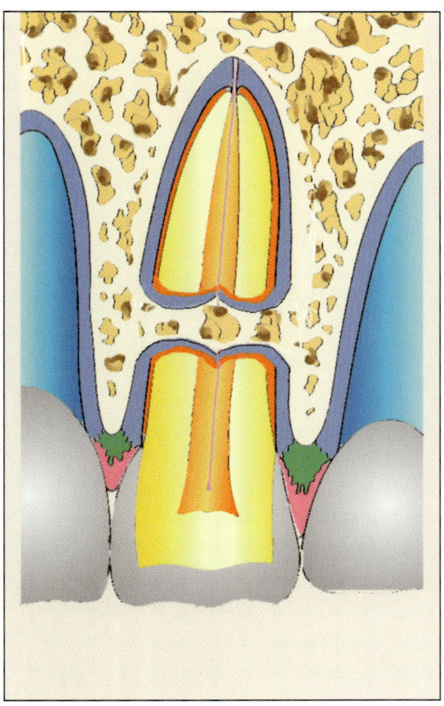

Fig 5-8c Healing with interposition of bone and connective tissue.

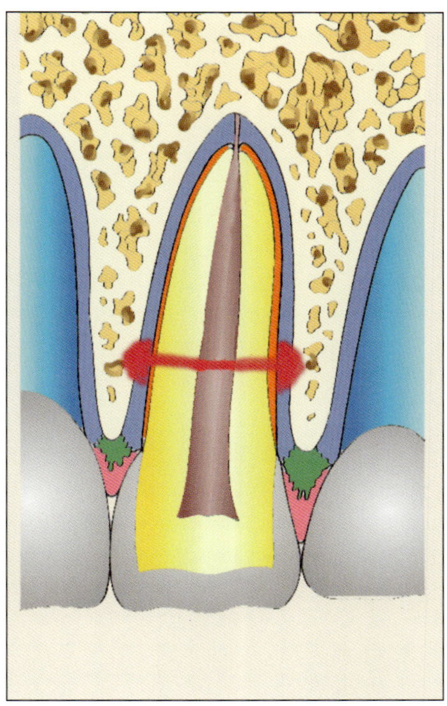

Fig 5-8d Lack of healing with interposition of granulation tissue.

Fig 5-9 Repair mechanism of interposition of connective tissue

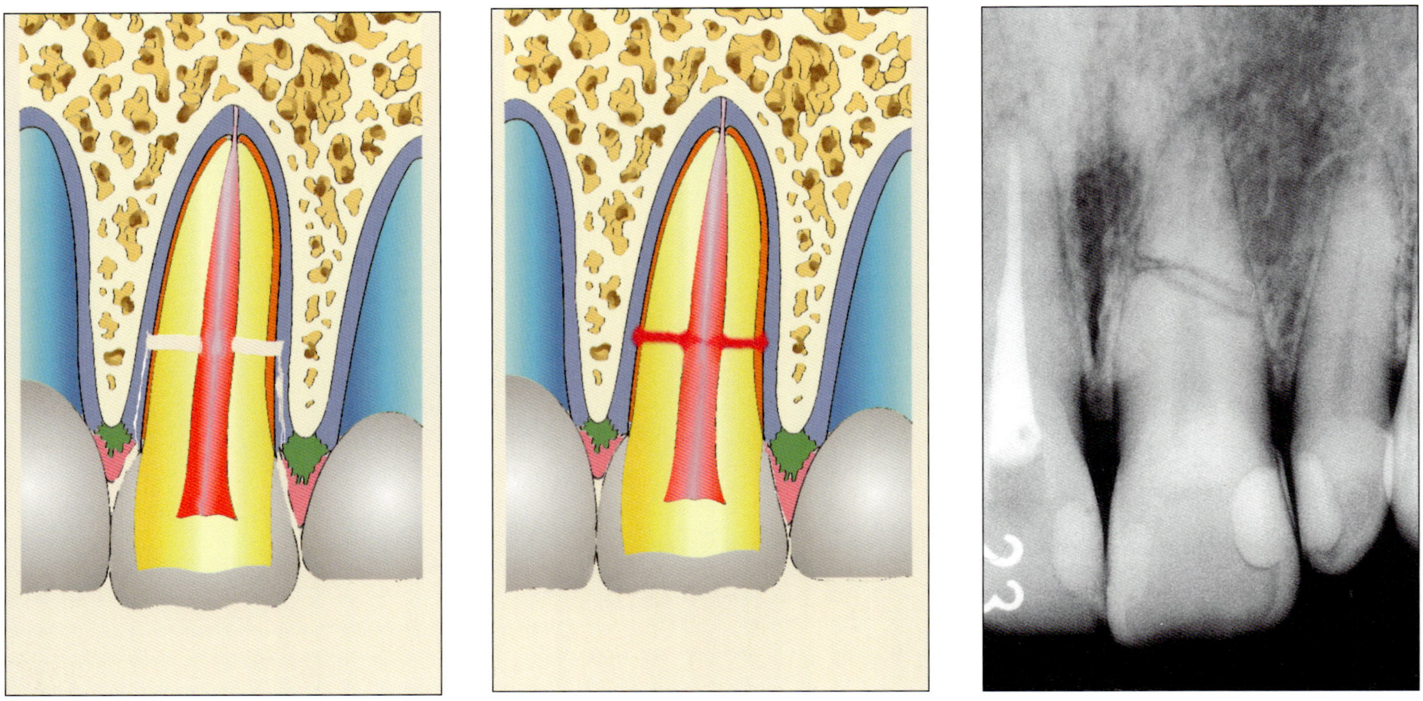

Fig 5-9a Root fracture with separation of coronal segment.

Fig 5-9b When fractured root segments are not properly repositioned before splinting, granulation tissue will develop in the blood clots occupying the open spaces between the opposing fracture surfaces. Areas of root resorption develop and periodontal ligament fibers form in these resorbed areas, resulting in healing with interposition of connective tissue. This common type of healing following root fracture can be seen radiographically as rounded edges at the site of fracture.

Fig 5-9c Healing with interposition of connective tissue. Note the rounding phenomenon of the root surfaces at the fracture site. The fracture line appears to be double because of the angulation of the fracture (the fracture is more coronal on one surface and more apical on the opposite side).

venting opposing root surfaces from joining by hard tissue formation, but instead connecting with fibrous tissues. This is recognized radiographically as rounded edges at the fracture site. Periodontal ligament fibers occupy some of the spaces (Figs 5-9b and c).

Healing with interposition of bone and connective tissue (Fig 5-8c)

If root fracture occurs early in development, especially during eruption, and if the wound is healed by the interposition of connective tissue, only the coronal tooth segment will continue to erupt. Consequently, bone invades the space between the tooth fragments. This is healing with interposition of bone and connective tissue[7] (see Fig 5-5g).

Interposition of granulation tissue without healing (Fig 5-8d)

Interposition of granulation tissue is the result of pulp necrosis (see Fig 5-7b). This lack of healing is a pathologic condition of granulation tissue with an abundance of blood vessels at the fracture site. Unless the cause is removed (the necrotic pulp), the condition will proceed to bone loss and root resorption. There is usually swelling, percussion pain, and radiolucency of the bone at the fracture site. Endodontic treatment will enable healing to take place with regeneration of the periodontal ligament at the fracture site along with hard tissue deposition by cells from the periodontal ligament. The subsequent healing is usually by interpositioning of connective tissue (see Figs 5-5i and 5-7c).

6

Concussion and Subluxation

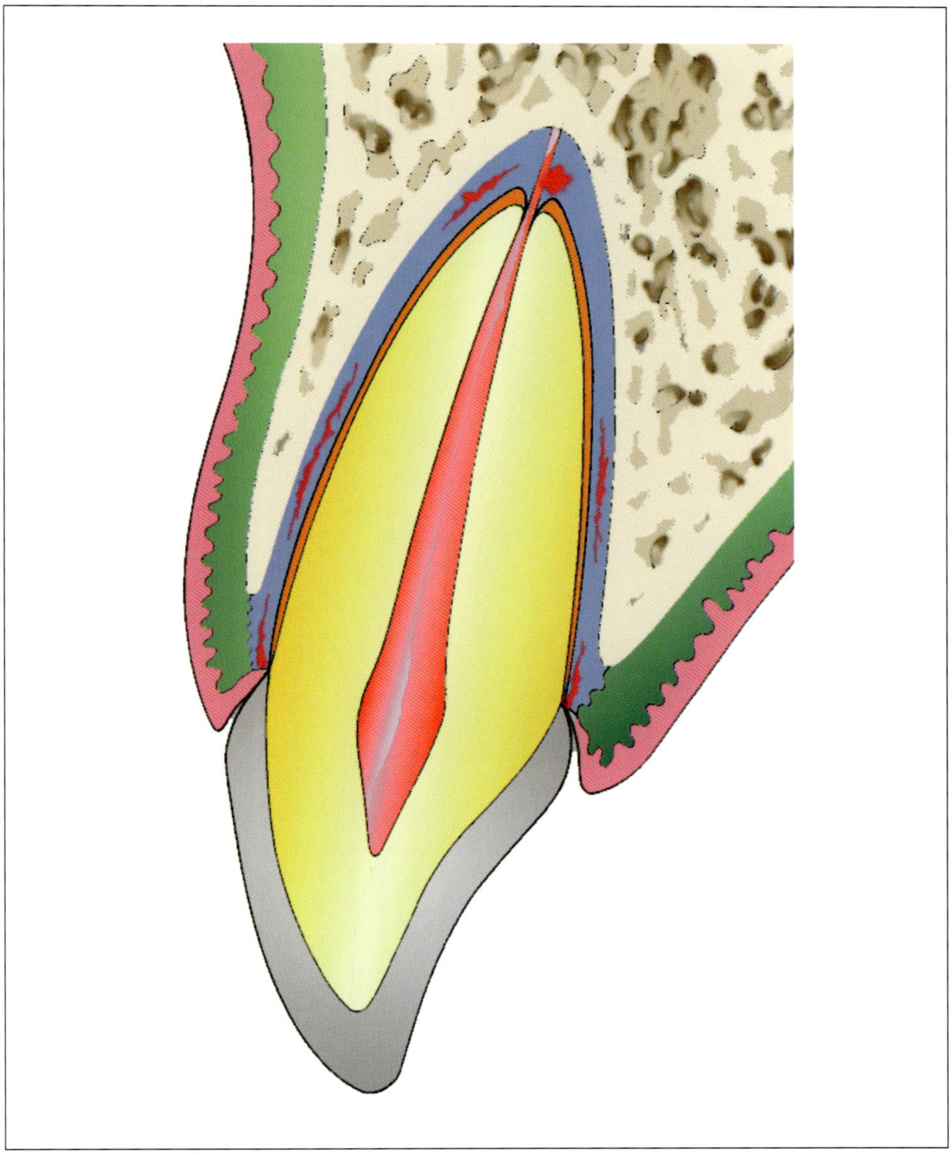

Luxation injuries involve trauma to the supporting tissues of a tooth. In increasing order of severity, luxation injuries are:

- Concussion
- Subluxation
- Extrusive luxation
- Lateral luxation
- Intrusive luxation

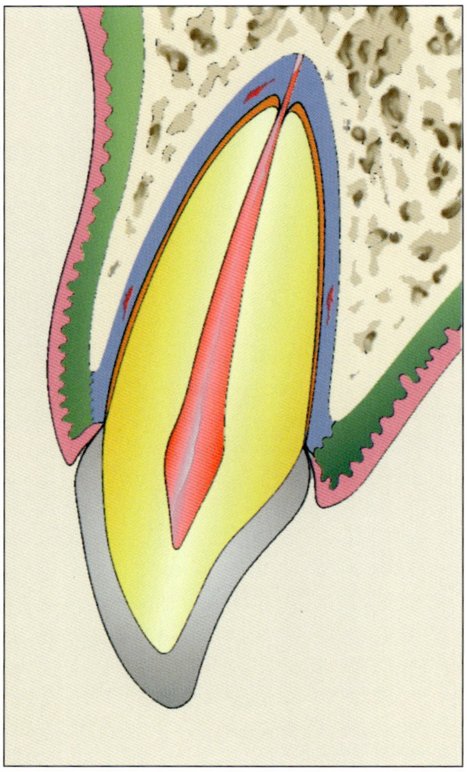

Fig 6-1 Concussion.

Common to all these types of injuries are varying degrees of trauma to the pulp, periodontal ligament (PDL), and surrounding alveolar bone and soft tissues. Consideration must be given to all of these tissues, in addition to the tooth, to develop proper treatment plans both for the acute aspect of the injury as well as for the long-term outcome. In this chapter, the two less-severe types of injuries, concussion and subluxation, are discussed.

Description

Concussion

Concussion is a minor injury to the periodontal tissues without malposition or mobility of the teeth. The blood supply to the pulp is rarely affected (Fig 6-1).

Subluxation

Subluxation results from injury to the periodontal tissues with a slight increase in mobility, but without malposition of the teeth. The blood supply to the pulp may be affected (Fig 6-2).

Examination and Diagnosis: Key Points

Without an obvious fracture or malposition of the teeth, there is a possibility of concussion or subluxation if there is percussion pain, slight mobility, or bleeding from the gingival sulcus. Concomitant with tooth fractures is often concussion or subluxation, which can affect the outcome (Figs 6-3 and 6-4).

It is important to check the vital response of the pulp with the electric pulp test (EPT). Even if there is no response, observe and check again because the lack of response might be temporary. If the periodontal membrane space is enlarged radiographically, there may be damage to the vascular system apically. The possibility of pulp necrosis is rare in teeth with immature roots, but mature, fully formed teeth develop necrosis often.

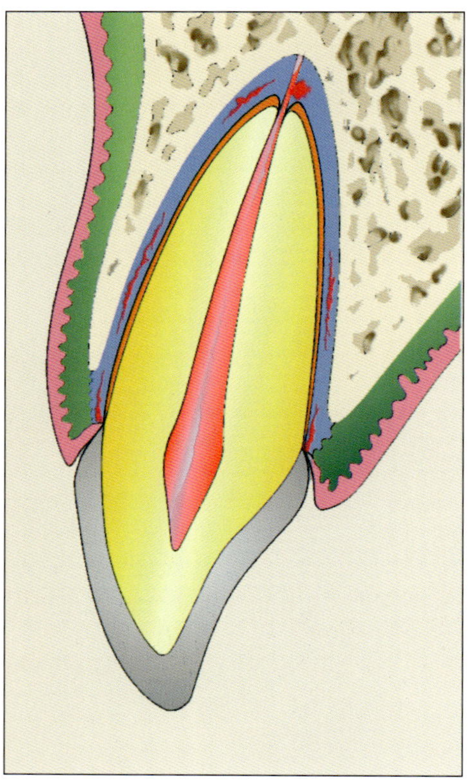

Fig 6-2 Subluxation.

Treatment Plan

Concussion

Only observation is necessary; monitor the pulp response periodically (Fig 6-3).

Subluxation

Usually only observation is necessary. Stabilize the teeth if the patient has problems chewing due to tooth mobility (Fig 6-5). Endodontic treatment is necessary if there are symptoms of pulp necrosis (Fig 6-6).

Fig 6-3 Crown fracture and concussion

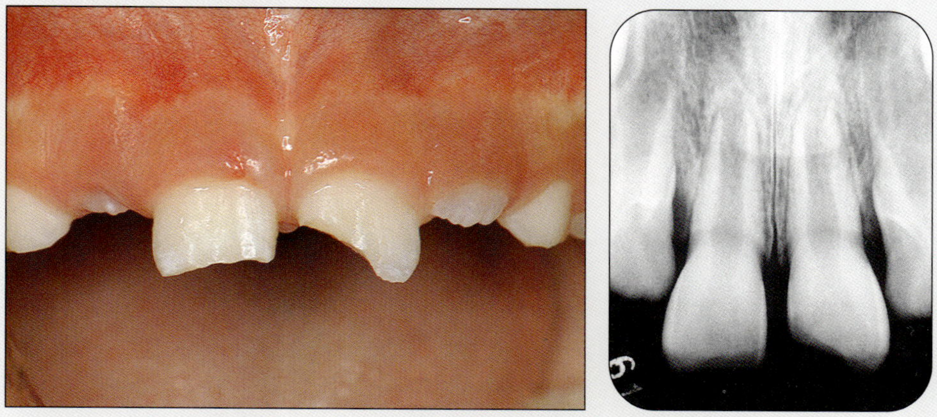

Figs 6-3a and b Preoperative view, 7-year-old boy with crown fractures of teeth 8 and 9.

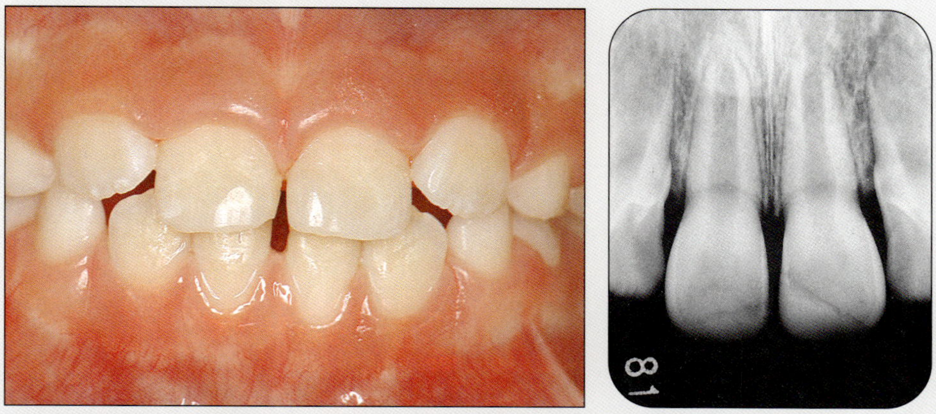

Figs 6-3c and d Three months after initial treatment. Note the slightly abnormal development of the apex of tooth 8. The Hertwig's epithelial root sheath was probably affected by the injury.

Fig 6-4 Crown fracture and subluxation

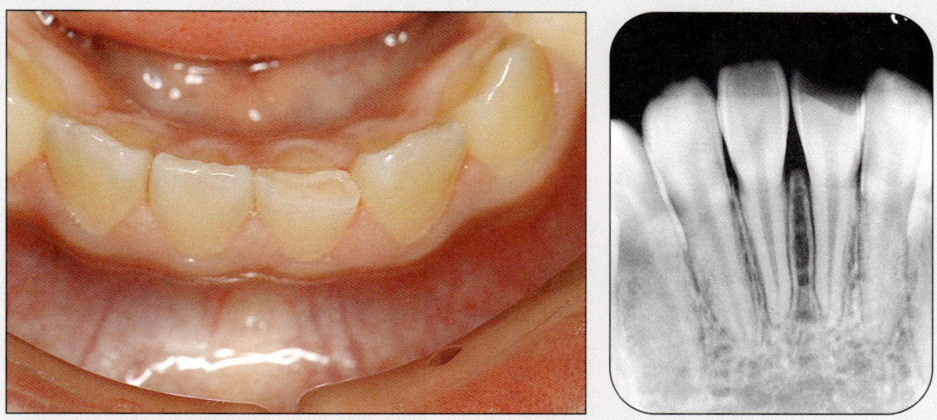

Figs 6-4a and b Preoperative view, 10-year-old boy with crown fracture of tooth 24.

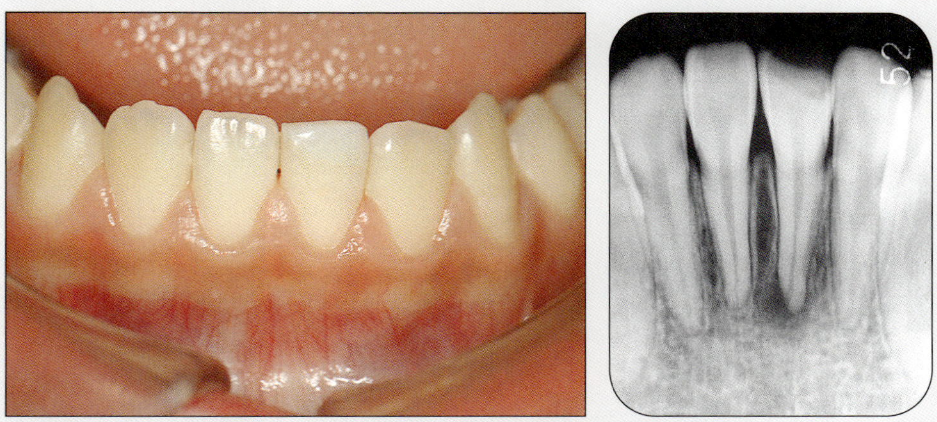

Figs 6-4c and d Three years after initial treatment. The pulp of tooth 24 has become necrotic due to the injury.

Fig 6-5 Treatment of subluxation, case 1

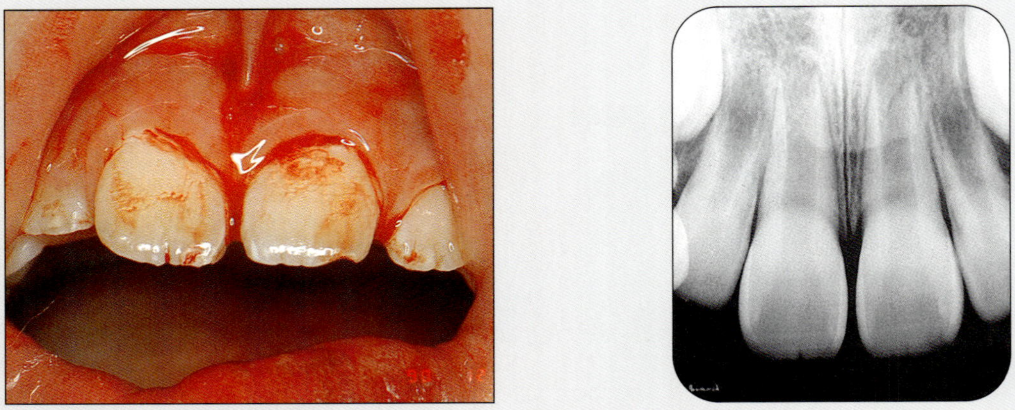

Figs 6-5a and b Initial examination, 6-year-old girl with subluxation of teeth 8 and 9.

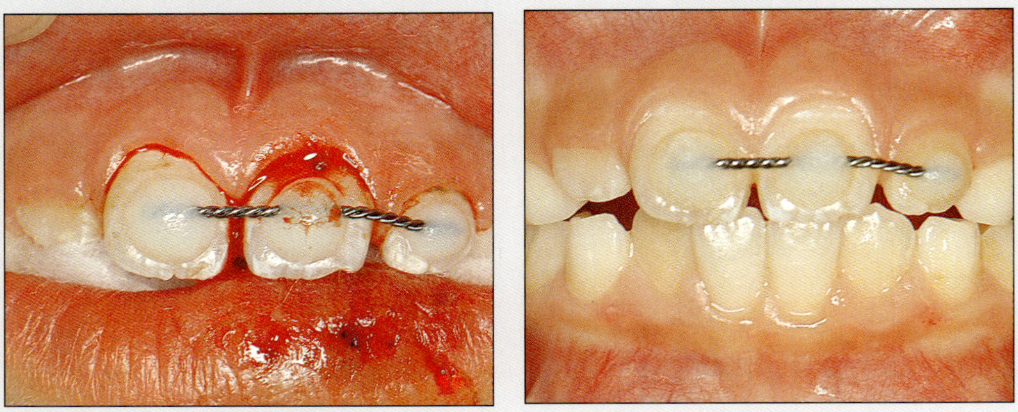

Fig 6-5c Immediately after splinting.

Fig 6-5d Two weeks after splinting before splint removal.

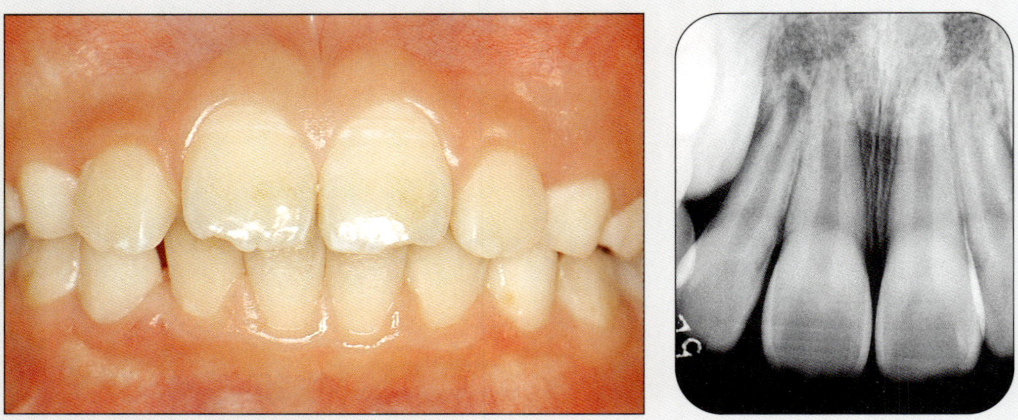

Figs 6-5e and f One year and 4 months after injury.

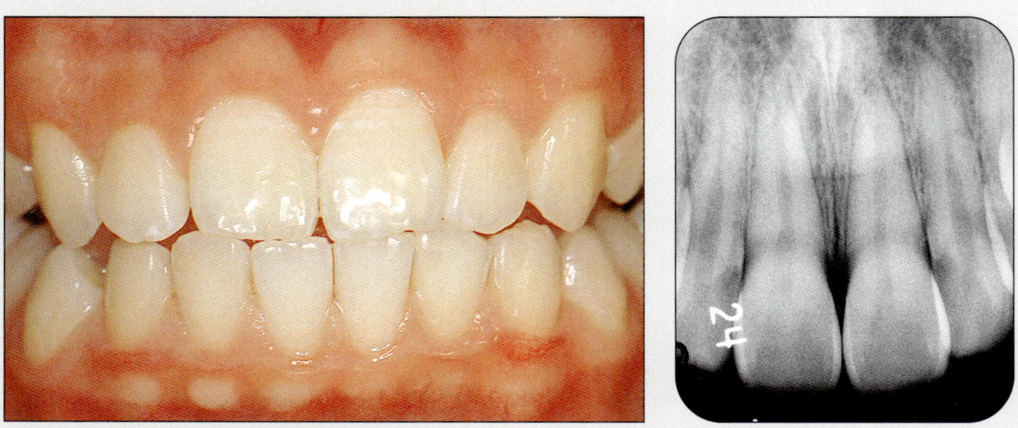

Figs 6-5g and h Approximately 6 years after injury. The patient is asymptomatic, and there are no signs of adverse effects of the trauma.

Treatment Procedures

1. *Examination and diagnosis*: Check for percussion pain, tooth mobility, existence and degree of bleeding from the gingival sulcus, and degree of trauma to the periodontal structures and the neurovascular bundle entering the pulp. Electric pulp tests and radiographs provide information about any detrimental changes (Figs 6-5a and b and Figs 6-6a to c).
2. *Splinting*: Stabilize teeth for 1 to 2 weeks if masticatory problems due to tooth mobility or pain occur (Figs 6-5c and d).
3. *Follow-up*: Monitor periodically for the development of pulp necrosis (Figs 6-5e to h and Figs 6-6d to i).
4. *Endodontic treatment*: Endodontic treatment is indicated when there is tooth discoloration, percussion pain, and indication of pulp necrosis based on the presence of an apical lesion. The initial endodontic procedure is to access the pulp chamber, remove the necrotic pulp tissue to the level where either bleeding is encountered or, if performed without local anesthetic, the patient feels some pain. Fill the prepared part of the canal with a calcium hydroxide preparation. These procedures can usually be performed without anesthesia. Follow-up observation is necessary (Fig 6-6i). Apexification is indicated should pulp necrosis occur to the entire pulp. After hard tissue closes the apex or the canal in the case of pulpotomy, complete the final root canal filling. In cases of tooth discoloration, bleach before proceeding with restorative treatment (Fig 6-7).

Apexification

Apexification is the process by which the open apex of a tooth with pulp necrosis and an incompletely formed root can be closed by deposition of hard tissue (probably cementum)[38–41] (Fig 6-8). To accomplish apexification, remove the necrotic pulp, clean the canal, and fill the canal with a calcium hydroxide preparation. After the apex is closed by hard tissue deposition, fill the root canal with sealer and gutta-percha (apical closure usually requires about 6 months). Figure 6-9 shows the mechanism of apical closure using calcium hydroxide.

Bleaching nonvital teeth

Bleaching is usually done before restorative treatment of nonvital, traumatized teeth. Pulp necrosis due to trauma tends to cause discoloration of teeth (Fig 6-6), and such discoloration appears to increase during apexification (Fig 6-7).

To bleach nonvital teeth, a mixture of sodium perborate and 3% hydrogen peroxide is placed in the pulp cavity for 1 to 4 weeks (Fig 6-10).[42, 43]

It is not necessary to change the bleaching agent during this time unless the tooth color does not change as desired. Bleaching can be enhanced by preparing the coronal cavity below the gingival level and removing the cavity smear layer with sodium hypochlorite.

After bleaching, glass-ionomer cement is placed to cover the gutta-percha, and composite resin is used to restore the tooth.

Fig 6-6 Treatment of subluxation, case 2

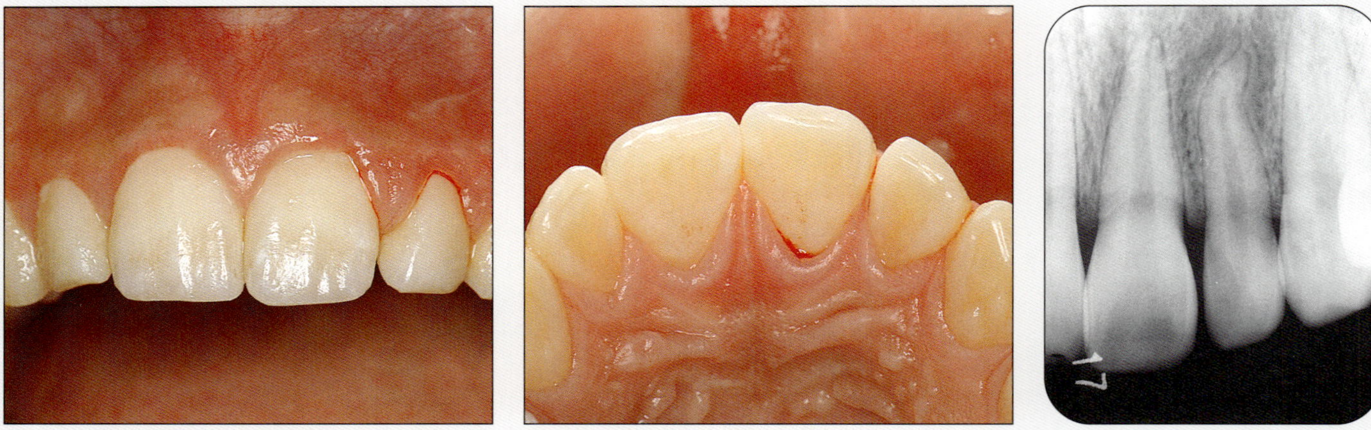

Figs 6-6a to c Initial examination, 14-year-old boy. There is subluxation of teeth 9 and 10 with no response to EPT.

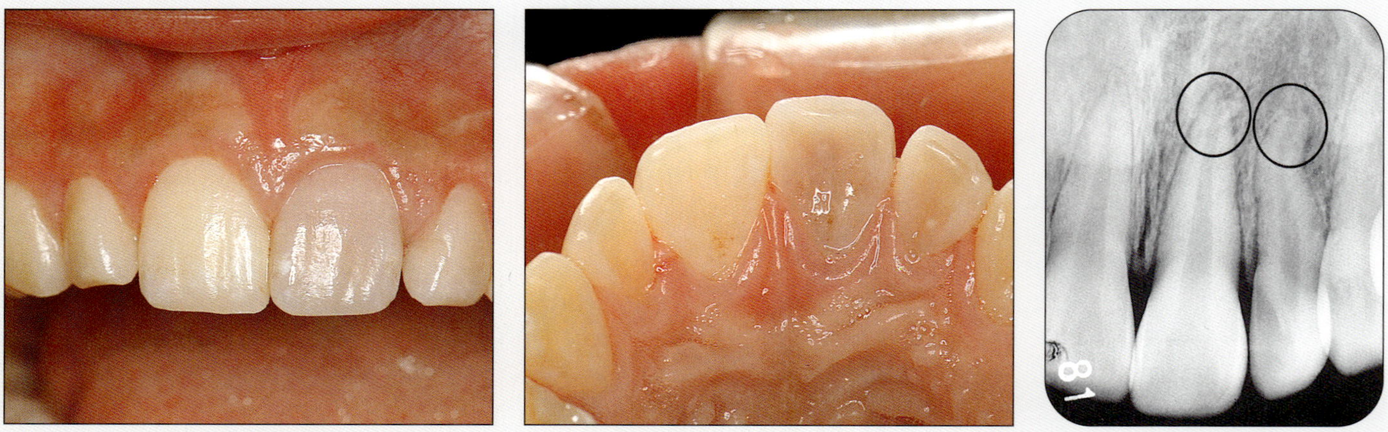

Figs 6-6d to f One month later. The crowns of both teeth are discolored. The radiograph indicates transient apical breakdown; compare the apical openings and note the wider apertures.

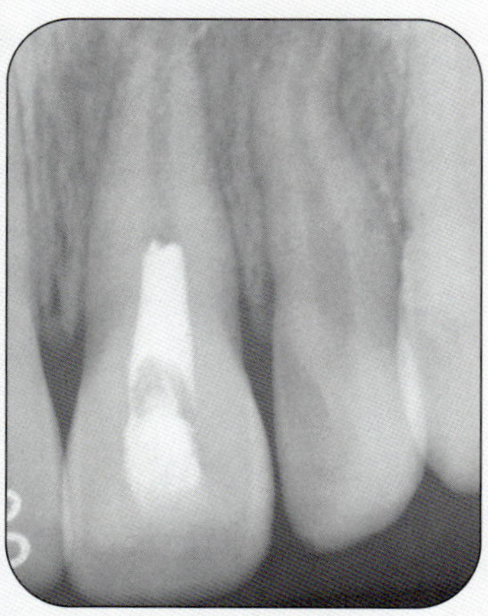

Fig 6-6g At 1 month, a decision was made to treat tooth 9 because of the severe discoloration. Only a pulpotomy was done, however, because vital pulp tissue was encountered in the middle part of the root. Tooth 10 was left untreated.

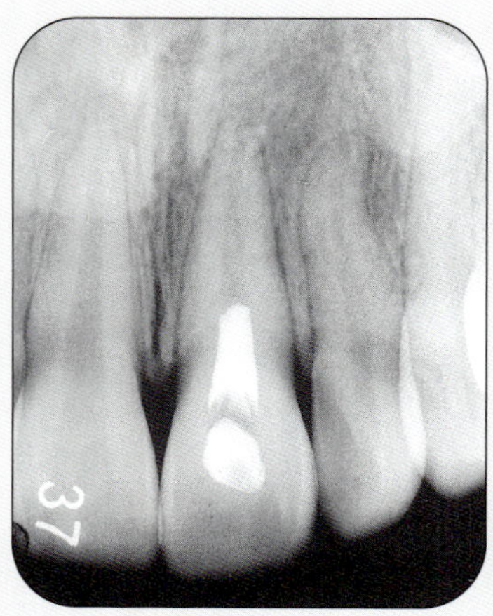

Fig 6-6h Five months after initial examination. Note the pulp obliteration in both teeth.

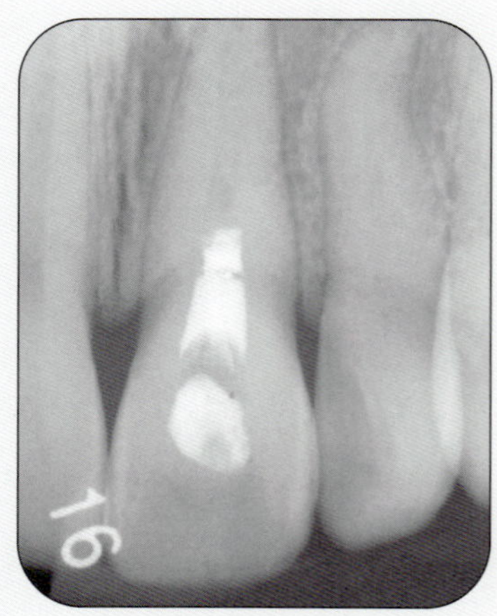

Fig 6-6i One year and 6 months after the initial examination. Pulp obliteration is very noticeable. Both teeth respond to EPT.

Fig 6-7 Treatment for subluxation, case 3

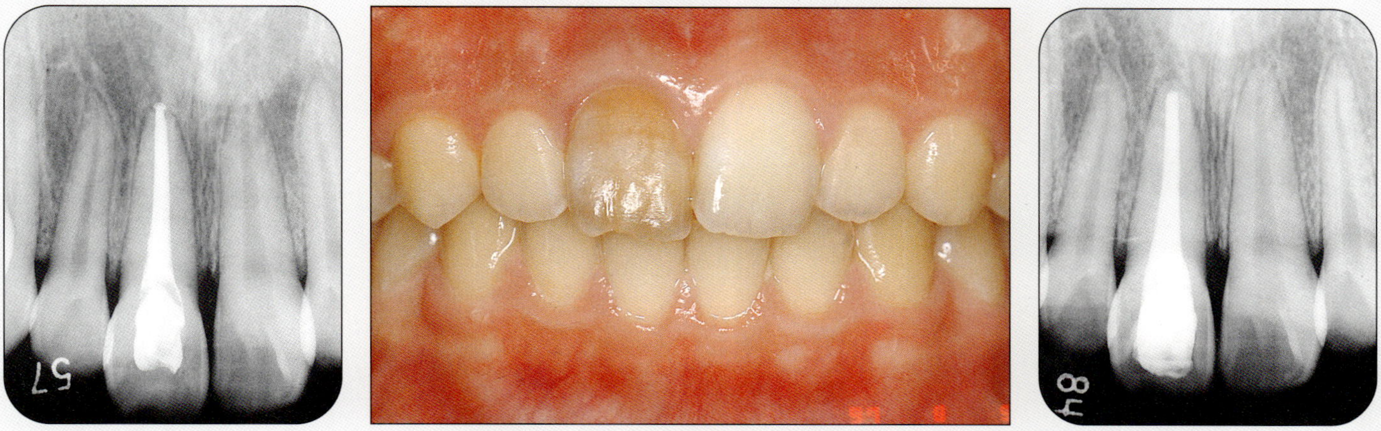

Fig 6-7a Twelve-year-old girl with a history of subluxation of tooth 8 undergoing apexification. Radiograph shows the beginning stage of apexification on tooth 8; the canal has been filled with calcium hydroxide. Note that the apex is open.

Fig 6-7b Ten months later. Note the discoloration of 8.

Fig 6-7c Radiograph taken immediately after endodontic treatment using sealer and gutta-percha. This procedure was done after confirming apical closure.

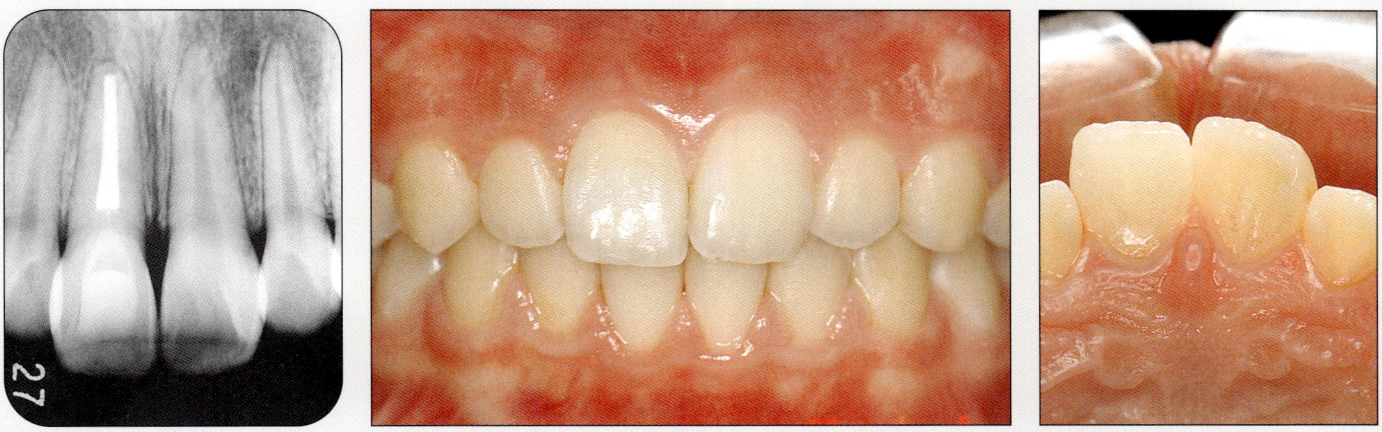

Figs 6-7d to f Sixteen months later. After bleaching the crown, restorative treatment was completed using composite resin.

Discoloration of teeth and pulp canal obliteration

Patients often present with discoloration of anterior teeth and pulp canal obliteration. They may or may not recall any episodes of dental trauma (Figs 6-11 and 6-12). The discoloration and pulp canal obliteration are likely the result of injury to the vessels at the apex, caused by subluxation.[44] (For pulp healing after avulsion and transplantation, see Chapter 9.) This phenomenon is the rapid apposition of osteodentin into the pulp cavity, which occurs when the blood supply to ischemic pulp resumes.[45–47] There may be total obliteration (Fig 6-11) or partial obliteration (Fig 6-12) of the pulp canals. There may or may not be a response to the EPT. Even when there is no response to the EPT, endodontic treatment is not necessary if the patient accepts tooth discoloration and if there is no apical lesion. It can be difficult to enlarge the obliterated canal.

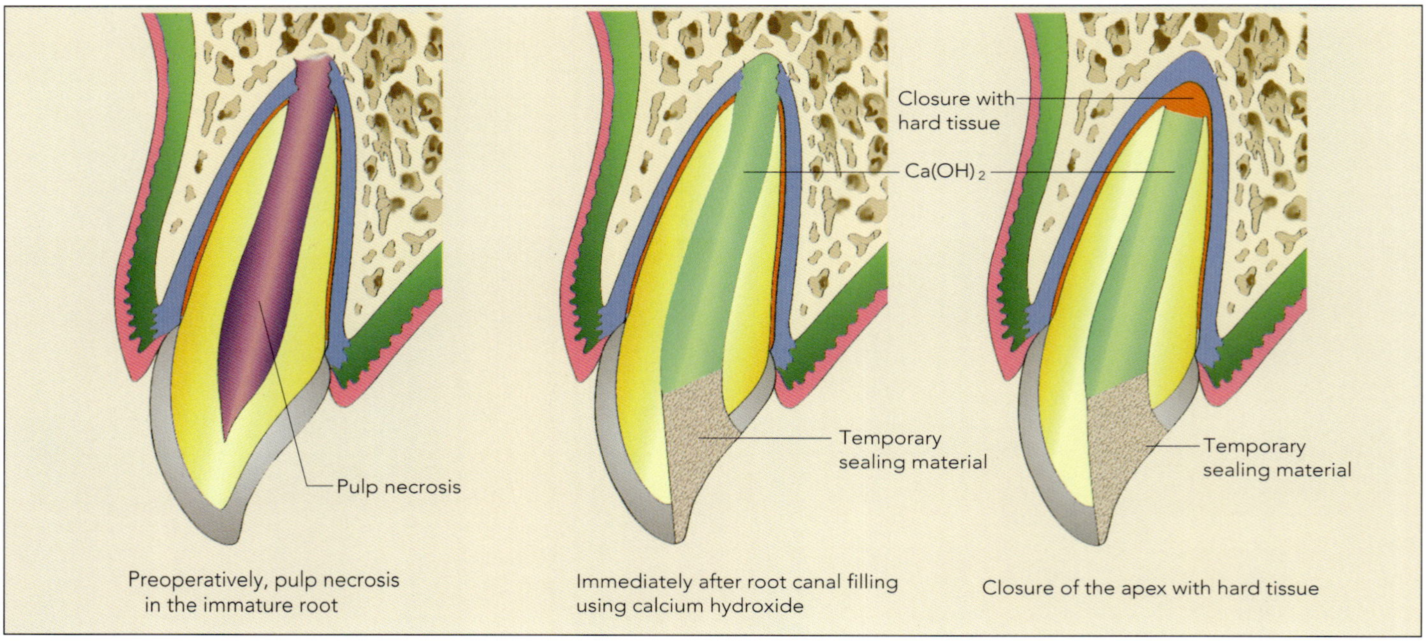

Fig 6-8 Apexification.

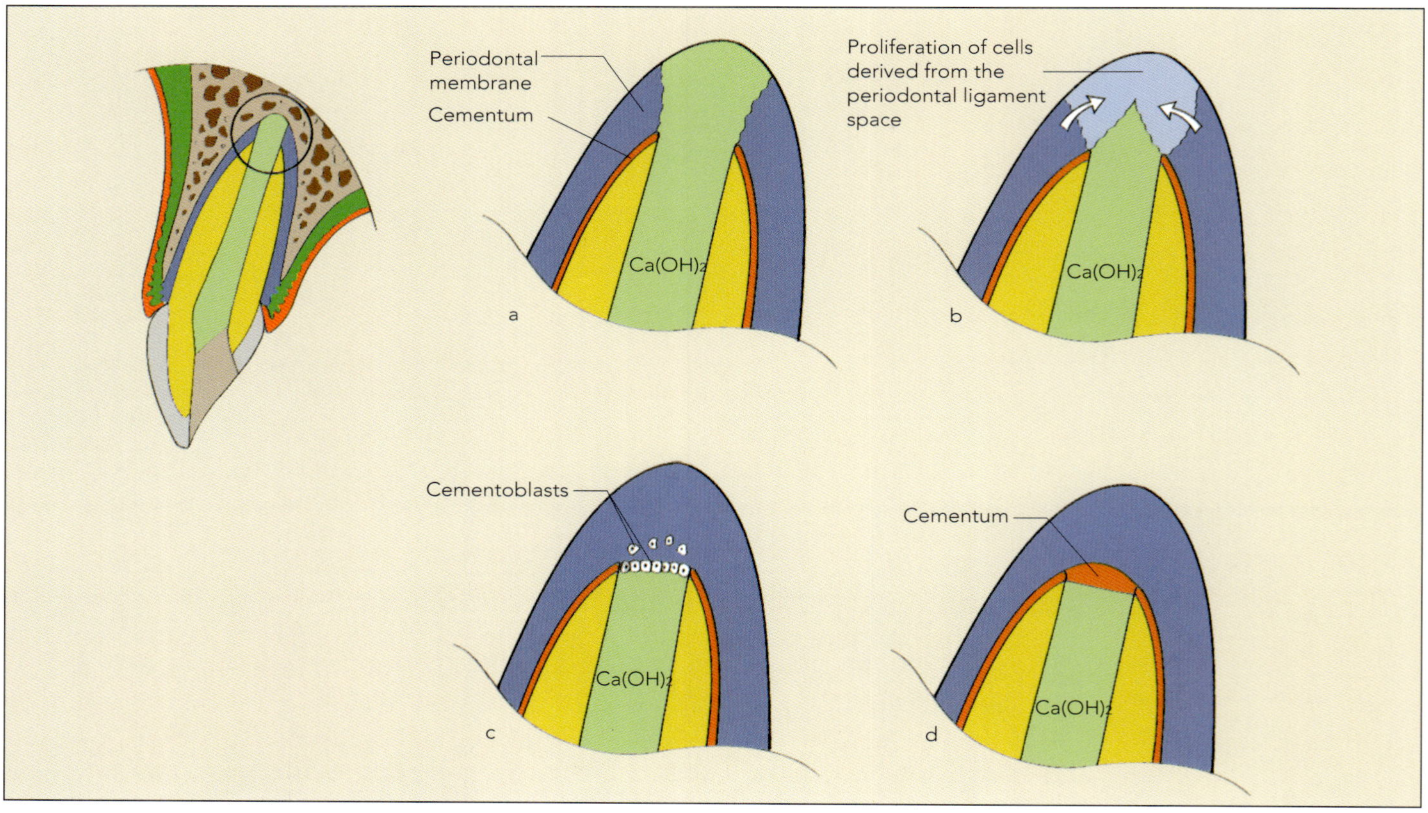

Fig 6-9 Healing mechanism of apexification.[22,41] (a) Immediately after treatment. Calcium hydroxide extruded through the apex causes degeneration or necrosis of the periodontal membrane and osseous tissue. Note the calcific deposit near the border of the necrotic layer and healthy tissues. (b) Approximately 1 month later. The necrotic layer and calcific deposit dissipate. Note the immature fiber and periodontal membrane tissue with an abundance of blood vessels around the apex. (c) Approximately 2 months later. Because cells have differentiated from the periodontal membrane (cementoblasts), there is hard tissue (cementum) apposition. (d) Three to 6 months later. The apex is closed by hard tissue deposition and is surrounded by periodontal membrane tissues. (Observation times are approximate.)

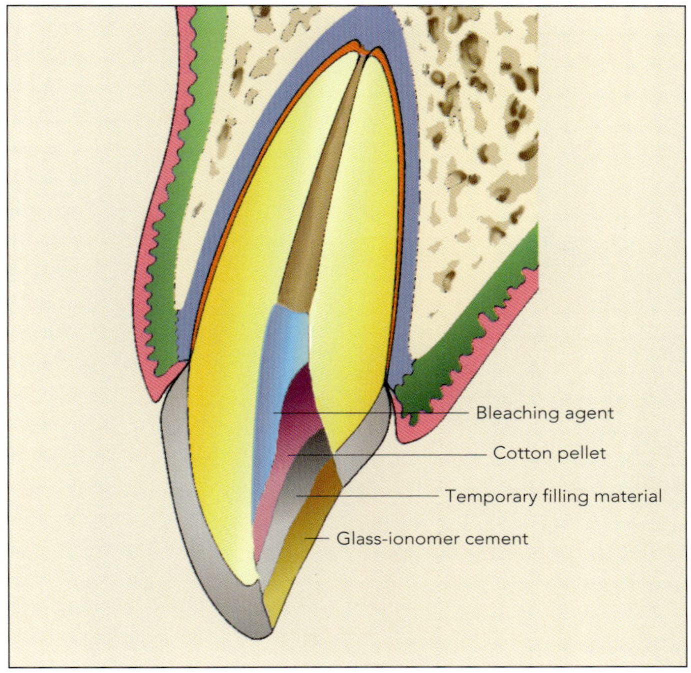

Fig 6-10 Bleaching nonvital teeth. Sodium perborate and 3% hydrogen peroxide solution are mixed immediately before bleaching. The coronal cavity should be prepared to below the cervical area (apically). Apply the bleaching agent to the entire surface of the facial dentin. Place a cotton pellet, temporary filling material, and glass-ionomer cement.

Fig 6-11 Tooth discoloration and pulp canal obliteration (total)

Fig 6-11a Thirty-six-year-old man. The tooth discoloration on tooth 8 is due to previous trauma (subluxation).

Fig 6-11b The pulp cavity is completely obliterated, and there is no response to EPT. However, there are no clinical symptoms, such as an apical lesion or pain on percussion.

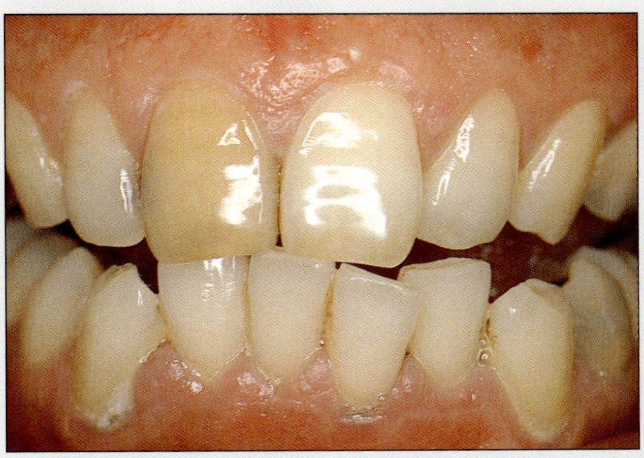

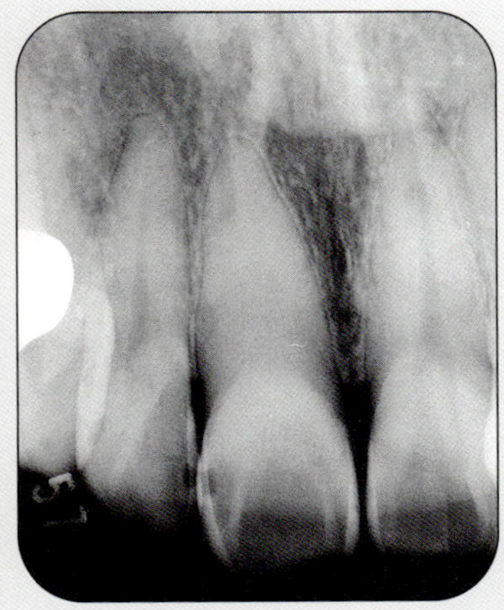

Fig 6-12 Tooth discoloration and pulp canal obliteration (partial)

Fig 6-12a Thirty-year-old man. The tooth discoloration on tooth 9 is due to previous trauma (subluxation).

Fig 6-12b Pulp canal obliteration is observed only in the root canal; the coronal pulp cavity is normal. The response to EPT is positive, and the tooth is considered vital.

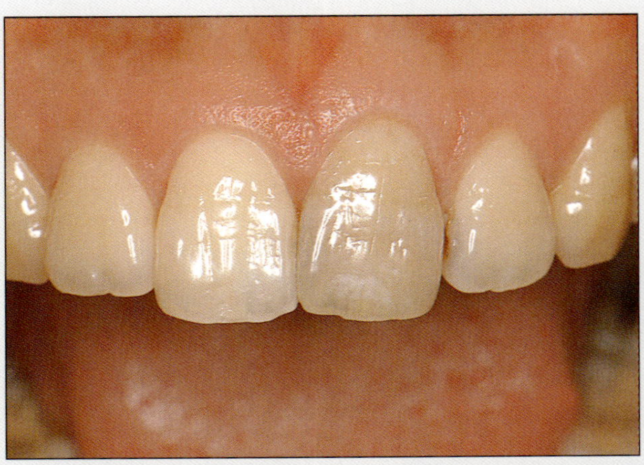

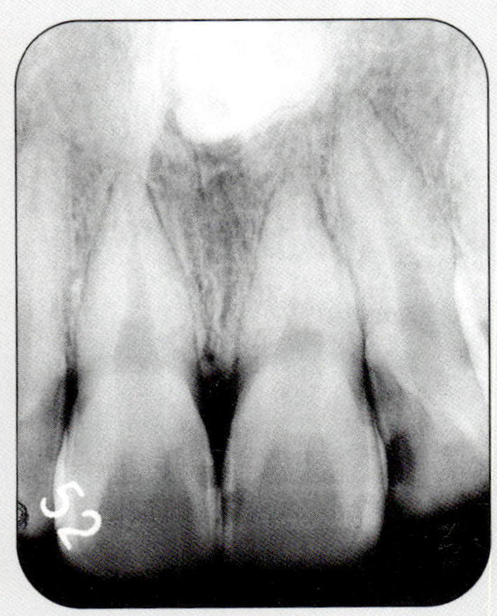

7

Extrusive and Lateral Luxation

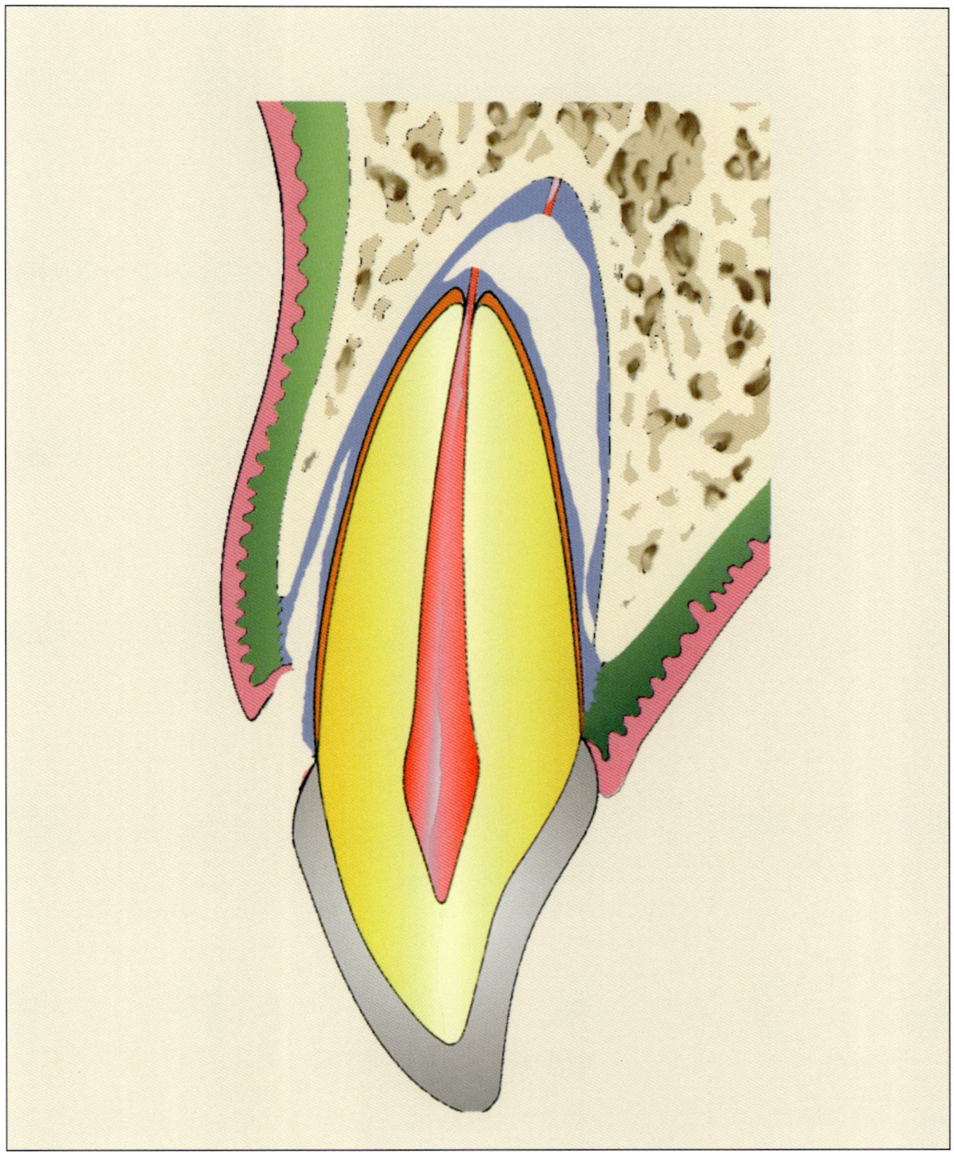

Extrusive and lateral luxations result in serious injuries to the supporting structures of traumatized teeth, along with severance of their apical blood supplies.

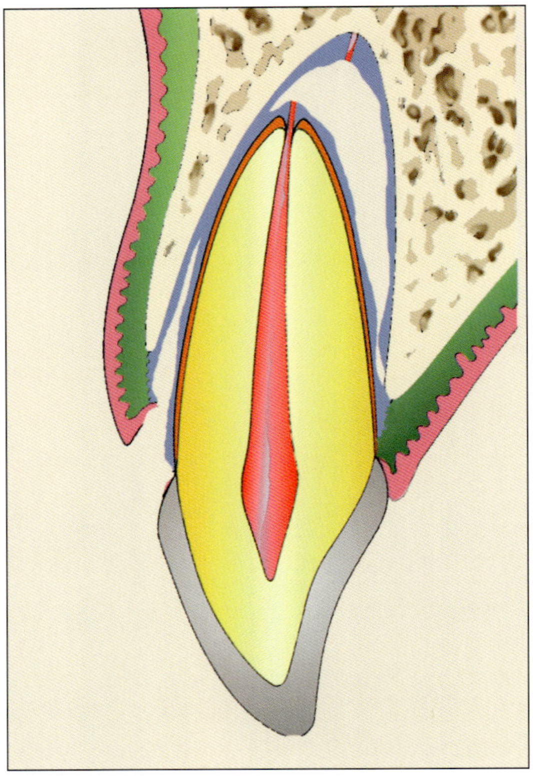

Fig 7-1 Extrusive luxation.

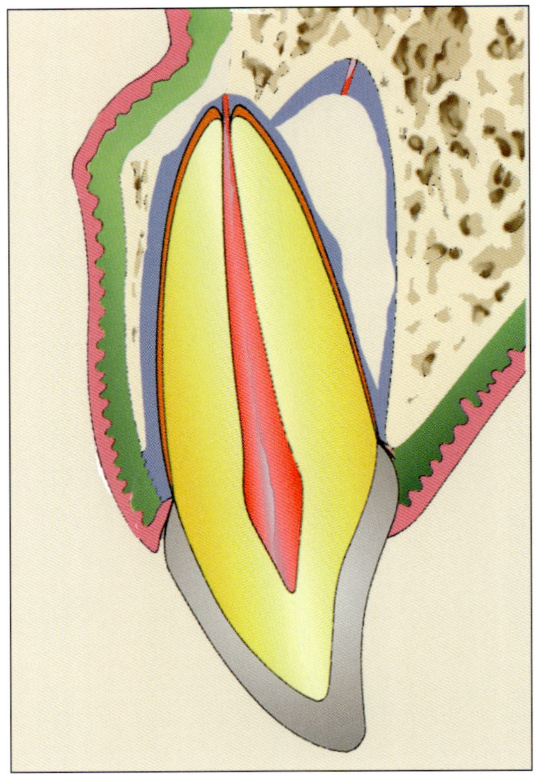

Fig 7-2 Lateral luxation.

Description

Extrusive luxation

An extruded tooth has been displaced coronally. There is partial separation of the periodontal ligament and often infractions of the alveolus (Fig 7-1).

Lateral luxation

A laterally luxated tooth has been displaced such that the coronal part of the tooth is often displaced palatally/lingually and the apical part of the root is displaced labially. Along with bony fractures and displacement, the periodontal ligament is partially severed (Fig 7-2).

Examination and Diagnosis: Key Points

Extrusive luxation is suspected when there is obvious malposition of the teeth and severe mobility, even without evidence of tooth fracture. Usually there is bleeding from the periodontal membrane and no response to the electric pulp test (EPT). In lateral luxation, the tooth is usually very firm in its displaced position. In both types of injury, there is enlargement of the periodontal membrane space evident radiographically.

Treatment Plan

For extrusive and lateral luxations, the treatment is repositioning, splinting, and observation. Endodontic treatment is indicated when there is no pulp healing (Figs 7-3 and 7-4).

Treatment Procedures

Extrusive luxation (Fig 7-3)

1. *Examination and diagnosis*: It is important to know the stage of root formation (Figs 7-3a to c) because pulpal healing may occur in teeth with immature roots (see Chapter 9, section on pulp healing).
2. *Repositioning and splinting*: After cleansing displaced teeth (Fig 7-3d), reposition them and use elastic wire and adhesive resin to splint to the adjacent teeth (Figs 7-3e and f). The splinting period is 1 to 3 weeks.
3. *Pulp treatment*: Endodontic treatment is indicated when there are symptoms of pulp necrosis. This should be performed 2 weeks after repositioning and splinting in mature teeth, and after observation in immature teeth (Figs 7-3g to i). In immature teeth that develop pulp necrosis, apexification is always the first choice of treatment (Figs 7-3j to m). Perform the final root canal filling after confirming apical closure (Fig 7-3o). Usually there is tooth discoloration (Fig 7-3n); therefore, after bleaching, restore the tooth with composite resin (Figs 7-4p to r).

Lateral luxation (Fig 7-4)

The treatment for lateral luxation is the same as for extrusive luxation except that the splinting period is 2 to 3 months. A longer splinting period is required because the alveolar bone fracture is complicated and takes time to heal. In lateral luxation, try to reposition the tooth while releasing the firmly wedged root apex. Special attention is needed to watch for transient marginal breakdown during healing (Fig 7-4g).

Fig 7-3 Treatment of extrusive luxation injury

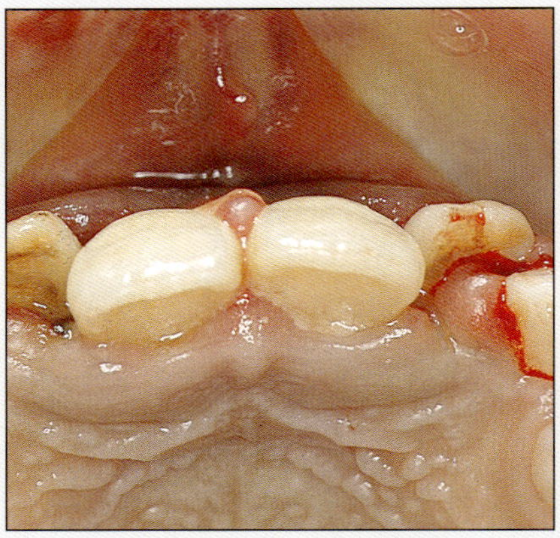

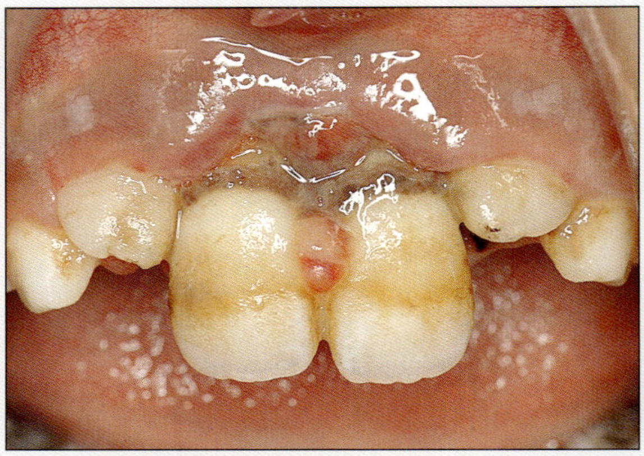

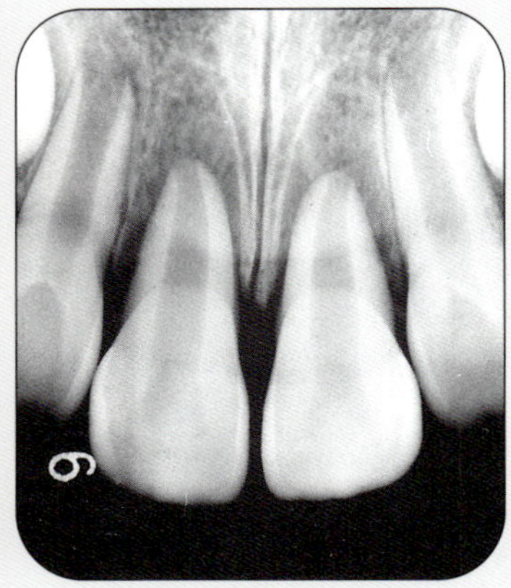

Figs 7-3a to c Preoperative views, 8-year-old boy. The initial visit was 1 week after the injury.

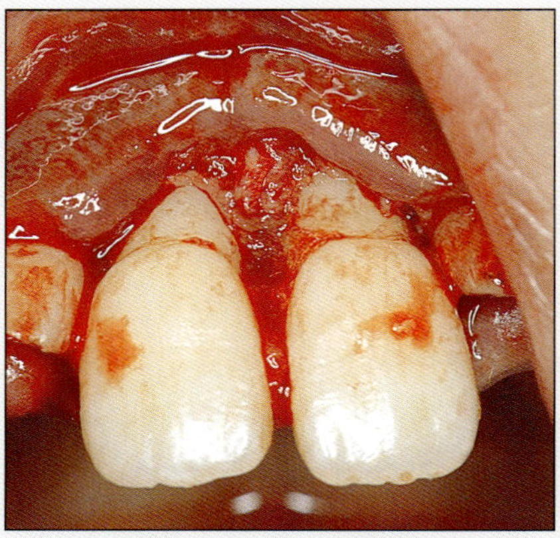

Fig 7-3d Debriding and cleansing of the extruded teeth.

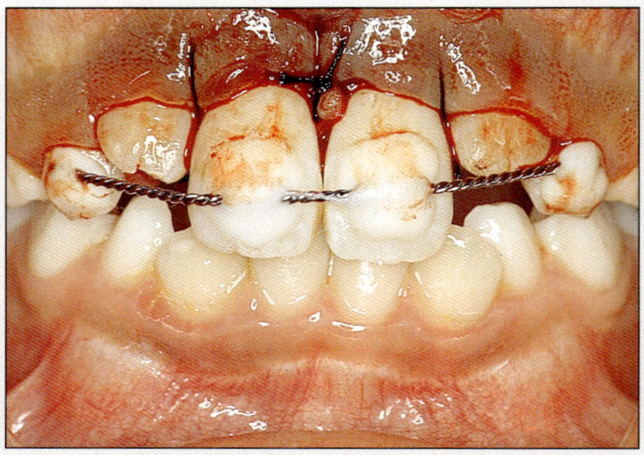

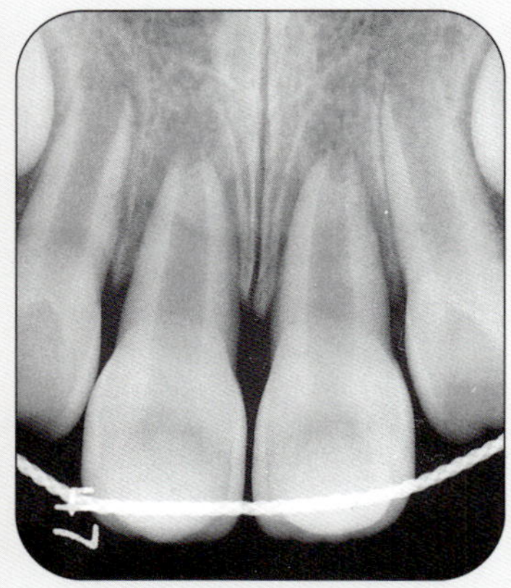

Figs 7-3e and f Repositioning and splinting. Complete repositioning to the original position was impossible because of blood clot formation in the alveolus.

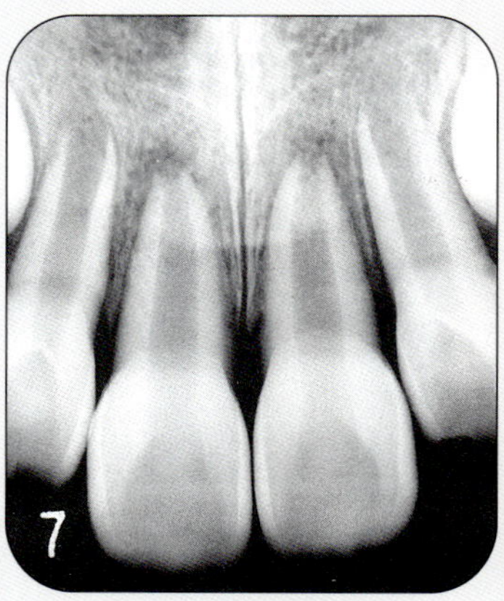

Fig 7-3g Forty-five days later.

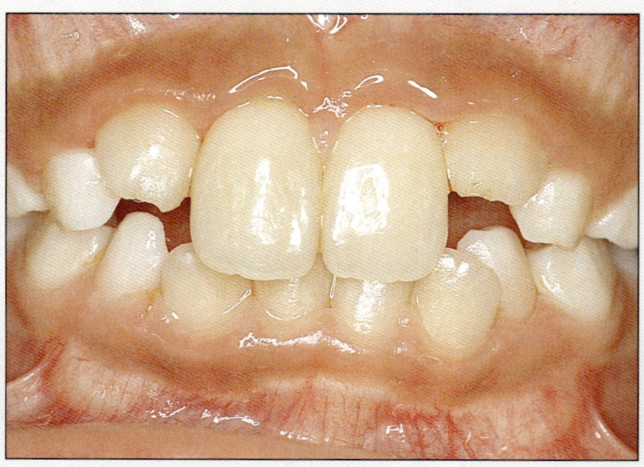

Fig 7-3h Four months later.

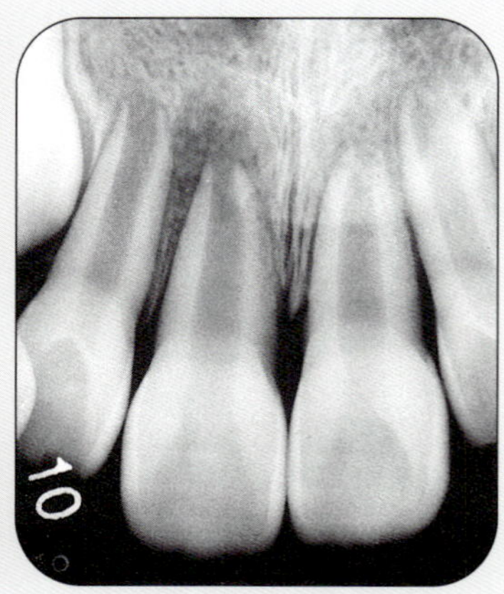

Fig 7-3i Five months later. Tooth 8 has percussion pain and an apical lesion.

Fig 7-3 (Continued)

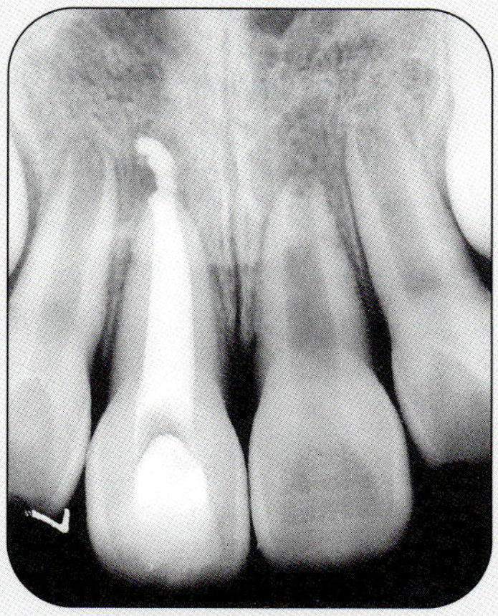

Fig 7-3j Radiograph immediately after apexification of tooth 8.

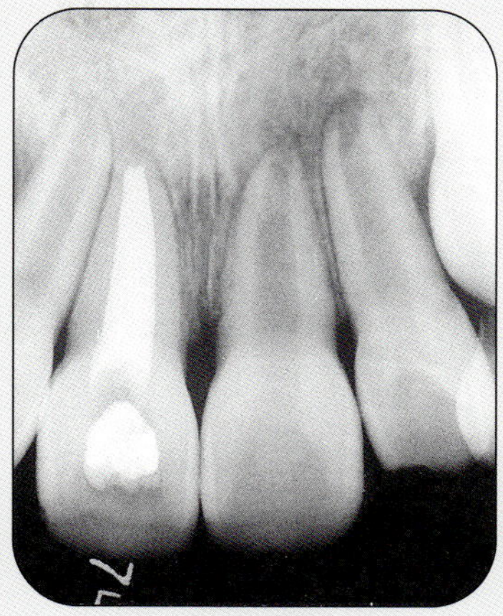

Fig 7-3k Eight months later (3 months after apexification). Tooth 9 has also developed percussion pain and an apical lesion.

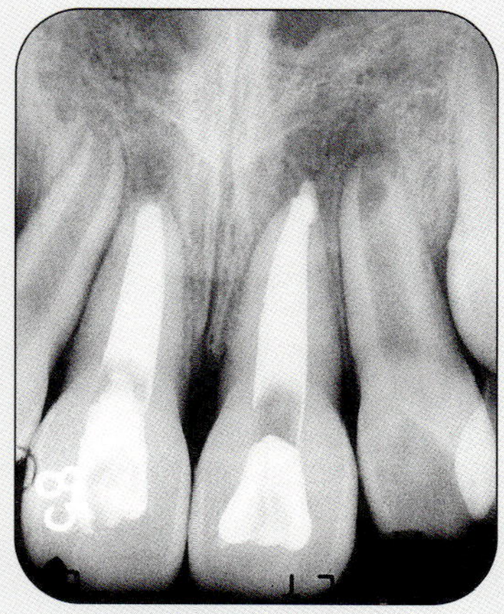

Fig 7-3l Radiograph immediately after apexification of tooth 9.

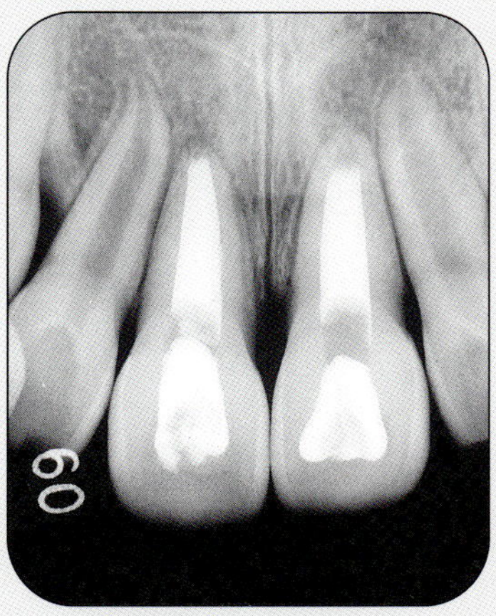

Fig 7-3m One year and 2 months later. The apexes of teeth 8 and 9 responded favorably to apexification.

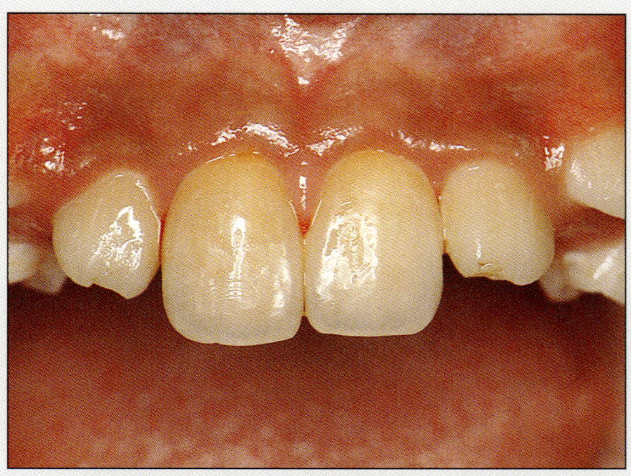

Fig 7-3n One year and 8 months later. Note crown discoloration.

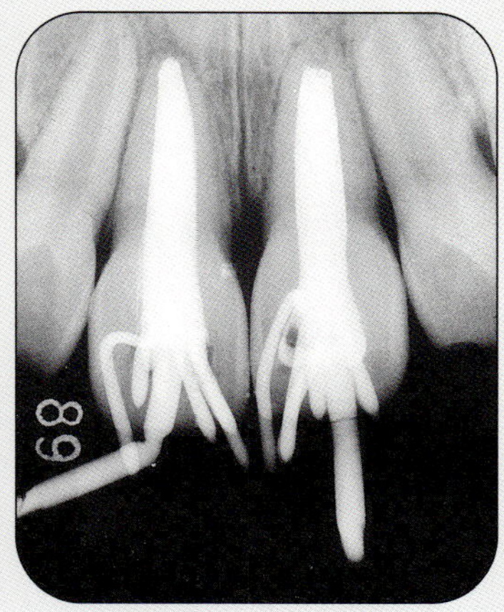

Fig 7-3o Radiograph after the final root canal filling with sealer and gutta-percha.

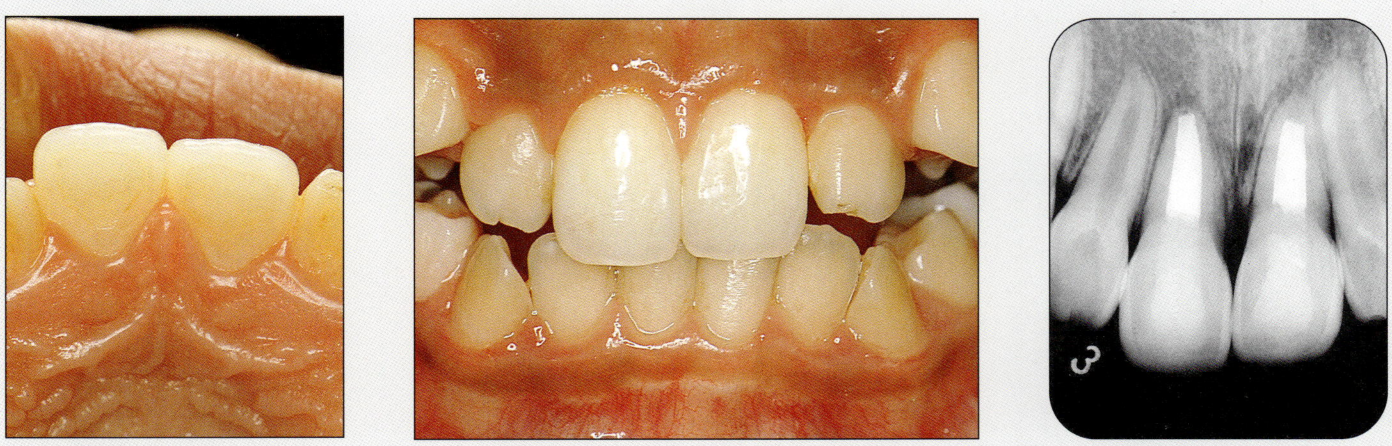

Figs 7-3p to r Two years and 7 months later. Bleaching of the teeth and composite resin restoration of the lingual access opening were completed about 9 months earlier.

Fig 7-4 Treatment of lateral luxation injury

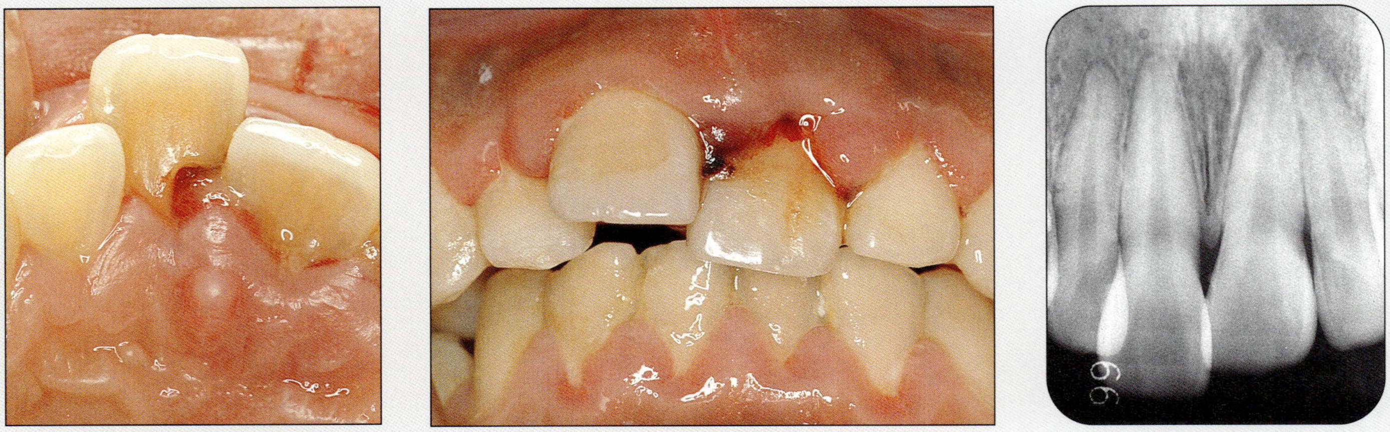

Figs 7-4a to c Preoperative views, 18-year-old man with lateral luxation of tooth 9.

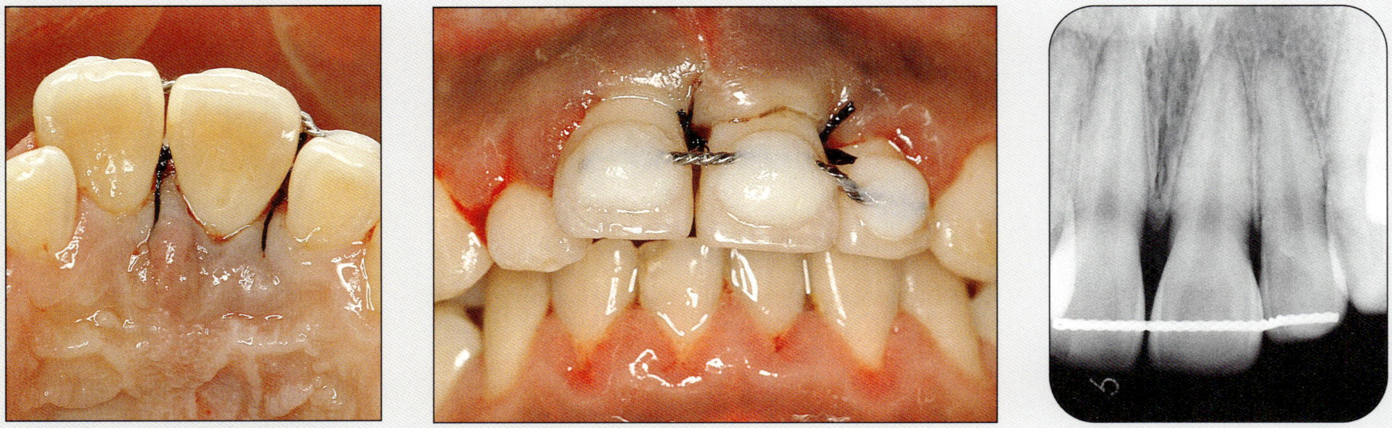

Figs 7-4d to f After repositioning and splinting.

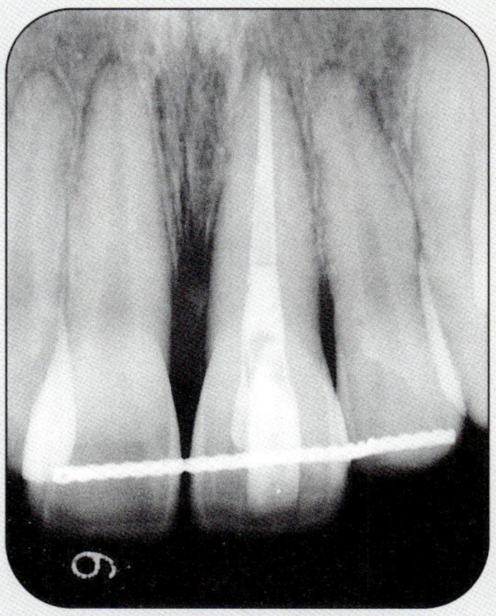

Fig 7-4g One month after repositioning and splinting. There is mesial cervical bone resorption on tooth 9.

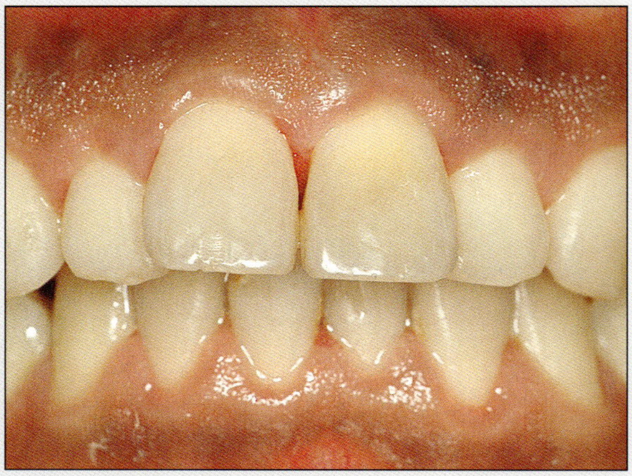

Fig 7-4h Five months later.

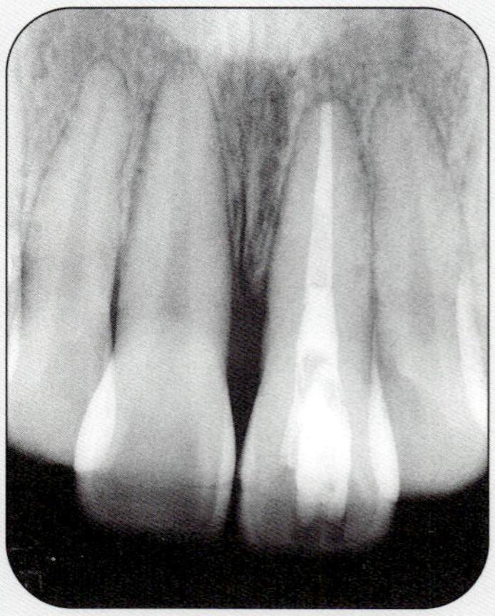

Fig 7-4i After five months. The resorbed alveolar bone is partially restored. A calcium hydroxide preparation was used for root canal filling and apexification.

8

Intrusive Luxation

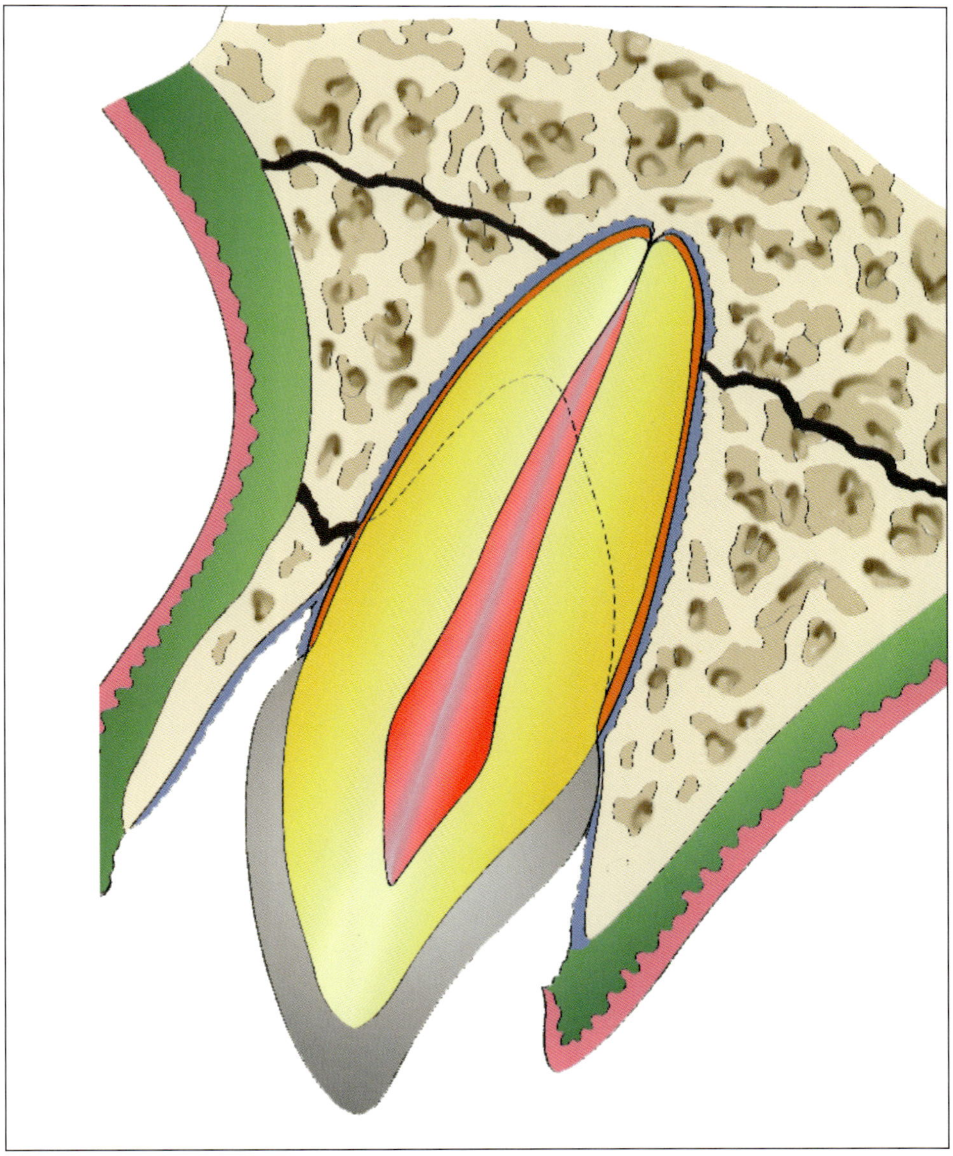

The treatment plan and procedures for intrusive luxation, considered to have the poorest prognosis of all dental trauma, are presented in this chapter.

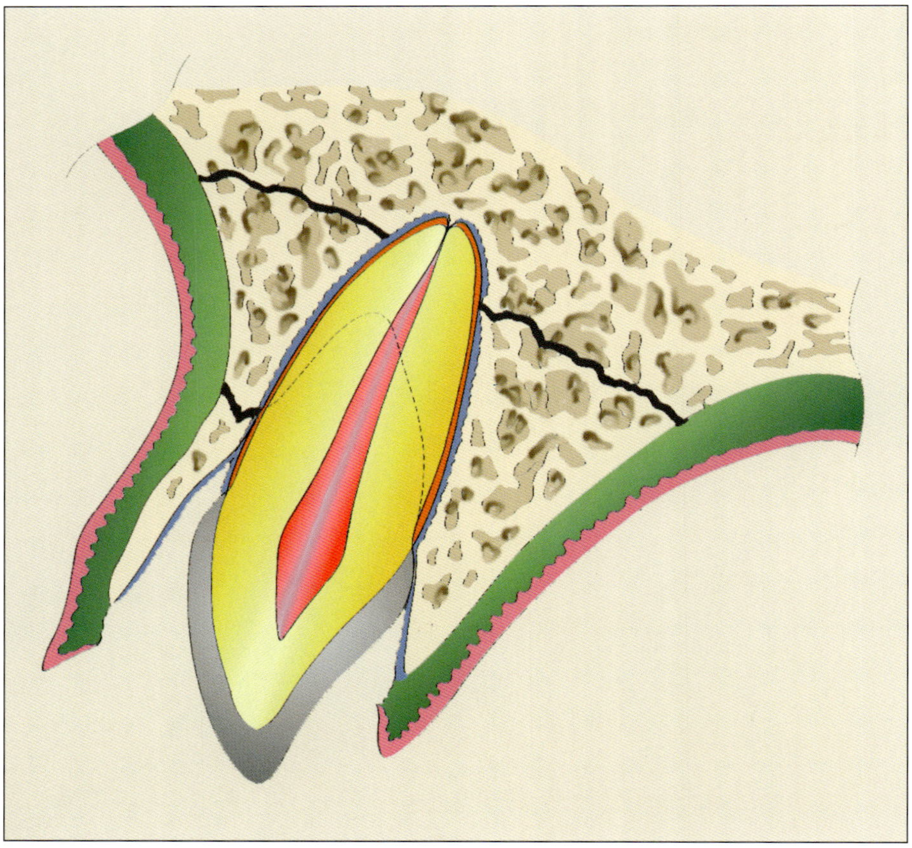

Fig 8-1 Intrusion (intrusive luxation).

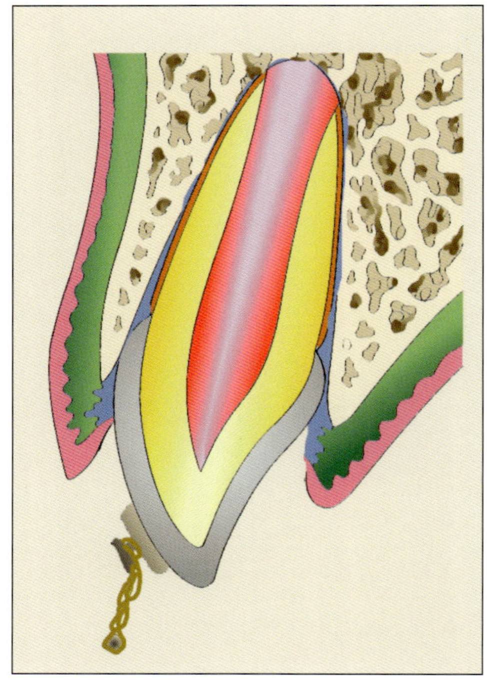

Fig 8-2 Orthodontic extrusion.

Description

Intrusive luxation is an apical displacement of the tooth. Fracture of the alveolar bone usually accompanies this trauma (Fig 8-1).

Examination and Diagnosis: Key Points

An intruded tooth can be displaced so extensively that it is no longer visible clinically. It may be mistaken for an avulsion, but the correct diagnosis can be confirmed by a radiograph. Intrusion is often part of more extensive trauma involving multiple teeth and fracture of the alveolar bone. In addition, there is extensive trauma to the periodontal ligament and the root cementum, resulting in a poor prognosis for the tooth. The intruded tooth is clinically very firmly implanted in the bone.

Treatment Plan

One possible treatment plan is orthodontic extrusion of the intruded tooth[7] (Fig 8-2). This can be done by raising a flap to partially reposition the intruded tooth and then placing a bracket for orthodontic treatment, which may begin about 1 month after the trauma. The author's preferred treatment plan for intrusive luxation, however, is surgical repositioning of the intruded tooth or transplantation of the tooth to the alveolus of an avulsed tooth lost in the same traumatic incident (Fig 8-3).

Fig 8-3 Treatment of avulsion by transplanting an intruded tooth

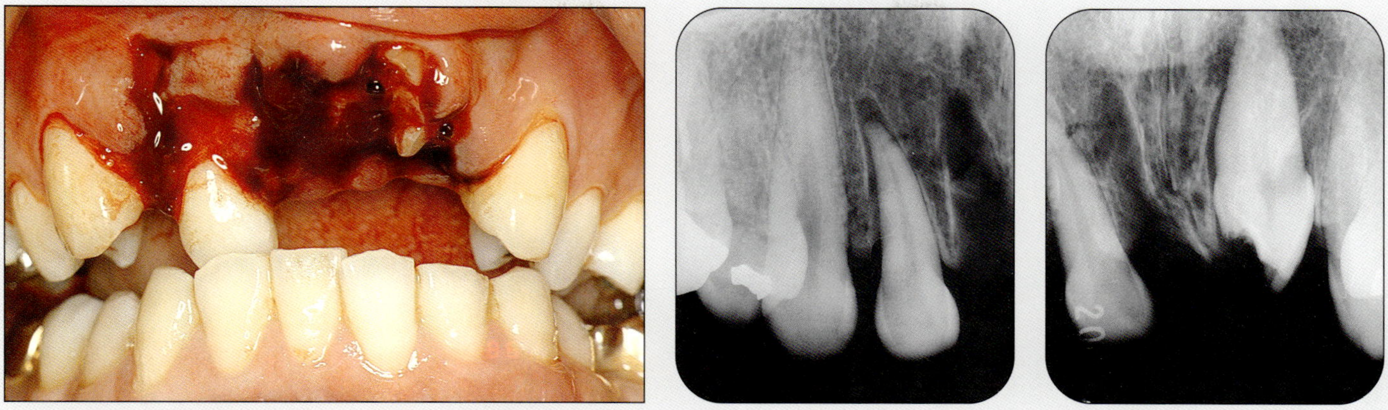

Figs 8-3a to c Preoperative views, 32-year-old woman. The initial visit is 3 hours after an automobile accident. Note the intrusive luxation of tooth 9 and the extrusive luxation with alveolar bone fracture of tooth 7. Teeth 8 and 10 are avulsed and lost.

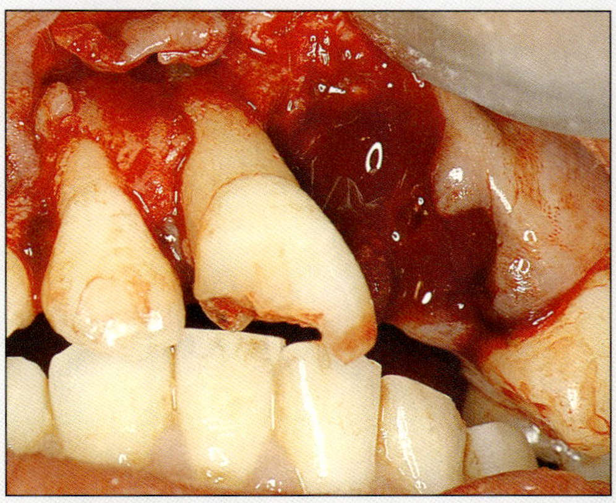

Fig 8-3d Repositioning of tooth 7 within the alveolar bone. The intruded tooth 9 is transplanted into the alveolus of missing tooth 8.

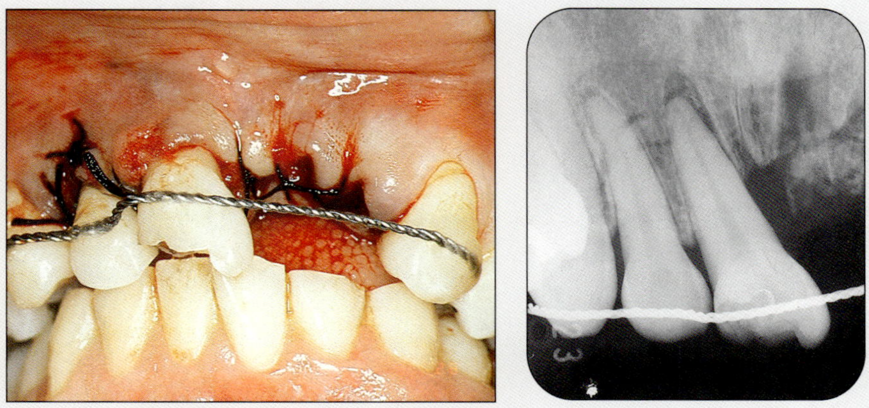

Figs 8-3e and f Immediately after repositioning, suturing, and splinting.

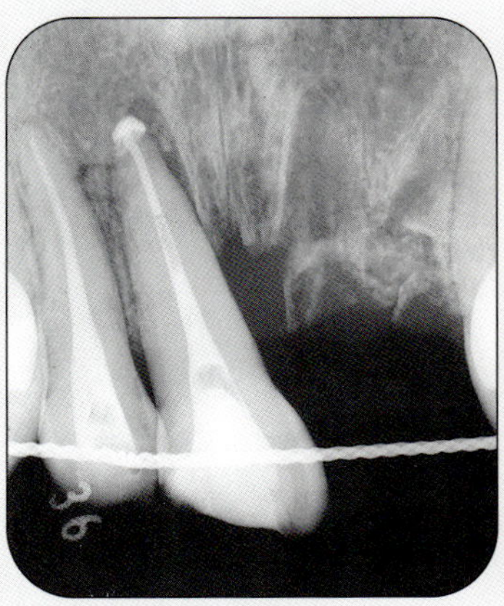

Fig 8-3g Two weeks later. Endodontic treatment of teeth 7 and 8 is performed with a calcium hydroxide preparation for the initial root canal filling.

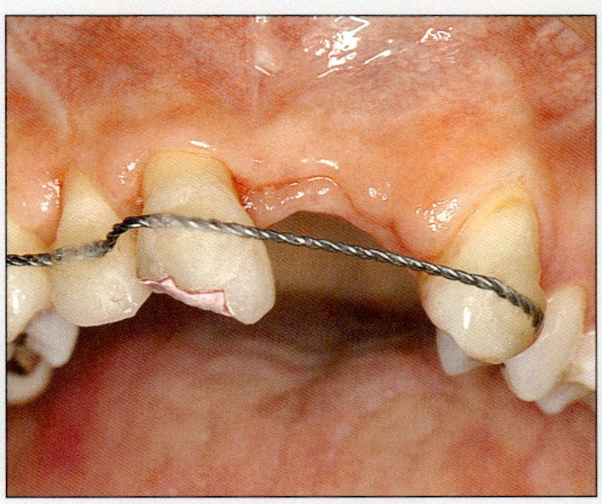

Fig 8-3h Three months later, before splint removal.

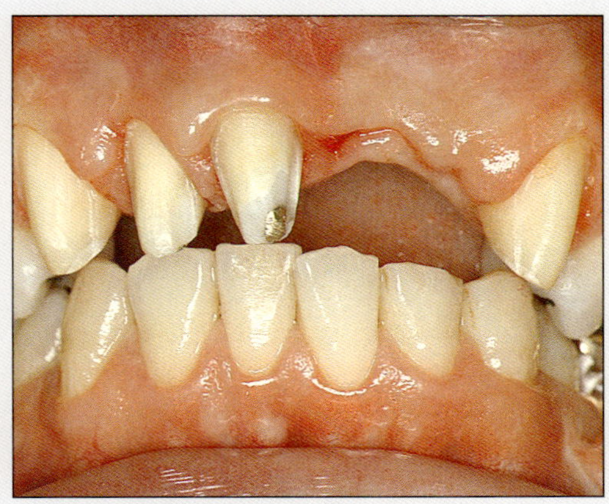

Fig 8-3i After tooth preparation for the fixed partial denture involving teeth 6 through 11.

Fig 8-3 (Continued)

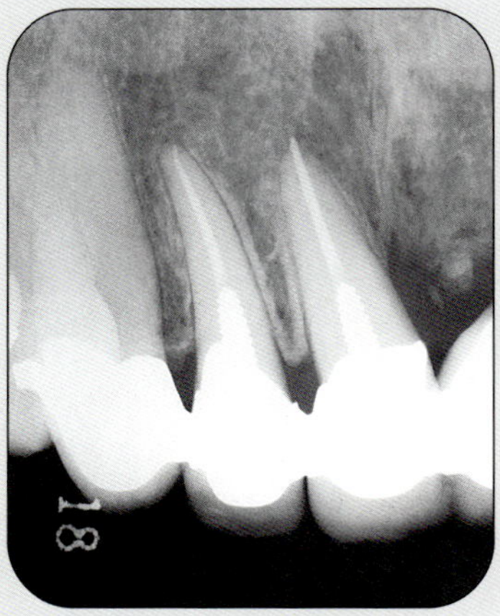

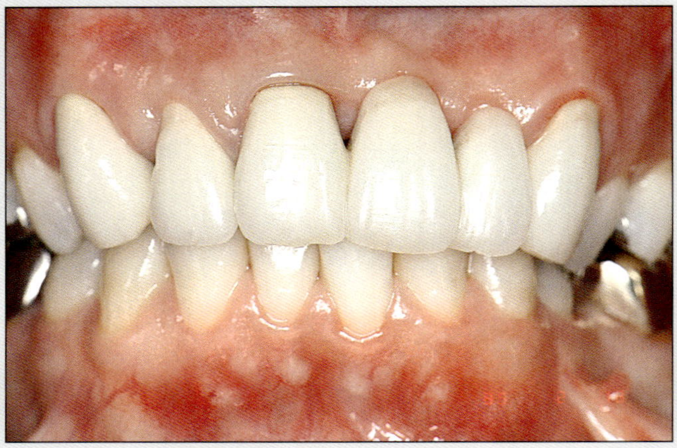

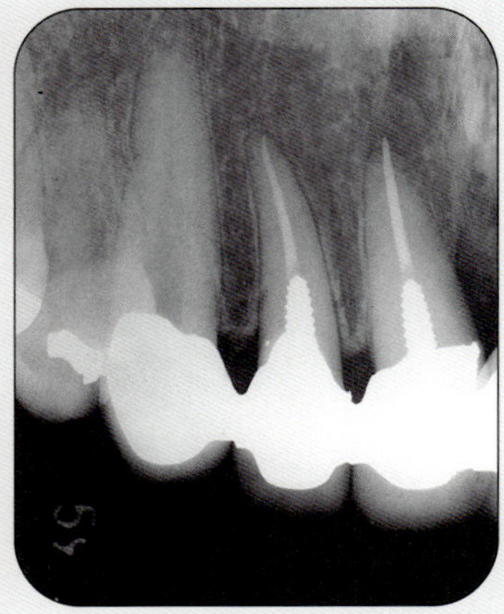

Figs 8-3j and k One year after initial examination.

Fig 8-3l Two years later.

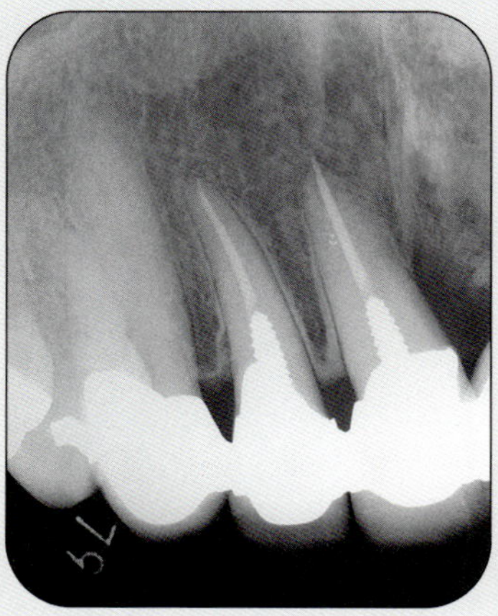

Fig 8-3m Four years later.

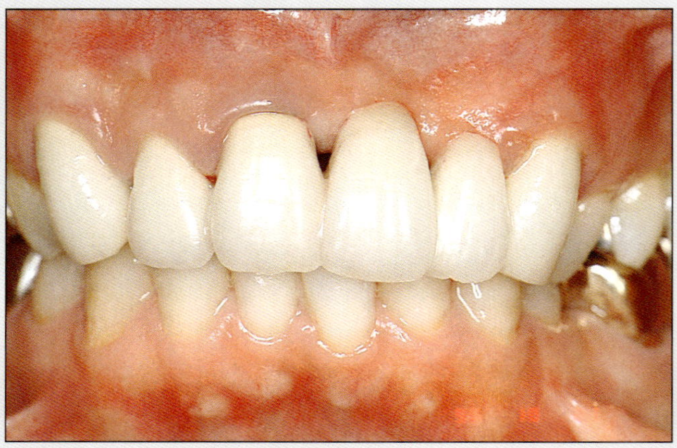

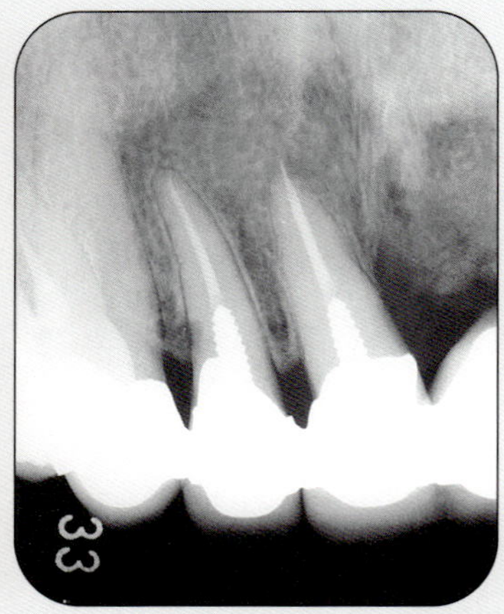

Figs 8-3n and o Ten years later.

Treatment Procedures

In intrusive luxation, treatment by orthodontic or surgical extrusion may not yield desirable results because of the severe damage to the alveolar bone around the intruded tooth. Therefore, if there is an avulsion of another tooth, it is possible to preserve the alveolar ridge and dentition by transplanting the intruded tooth to the alveolus of the avulsed tooth, where the alveolar bone may be more intact.

1. *Examination and diagnosis*: Recognize intrusive luxation and the degree of alveolar bone damage, in addition to other problems related to the trauma (Figs 8-3a to c).
2. *Administer anesthetic.*
3. *Transplantation of the intruded tooth*: Surgically transplant the intruded tooth into the alveolus of the avulsed tooth (Fig 8-3d).
4. *Repositioning and splinting*: Treat the problems related to the trauma and the alveolar bone fracture at the same time, and suture and splint (Figs 8-3d to f). Place a surgical dressing if possible.

5. *Endodontic treatment*: Perform endodontic treatment of the transplanted tooth or other traumatized teeth about 2 weeks later. Use a calcium hydroxide preparation for the initial root canal filling (Fig 8-3g).
6. *Follow-up and removal of splint*: Wait for healing of the fracture and transplanted tooth. Remove splint 2 to 3 months later if there are no problems (Fig 8-3h).
7. *Final endodontic treatment*: Use sealer and gutta-percha to replace the calcium hydroxide preparation.
8. *Prosthodontic treatment*: Perform prosthodontic treatment to restore esthetics and function (Figs 8-3i to k).
9. *Follow-up:* Re-evaluate at regular intervals to detect problems of the transplanted tooth and other traumatized teeth (Figs 8-3l to o).

9

Avulsion

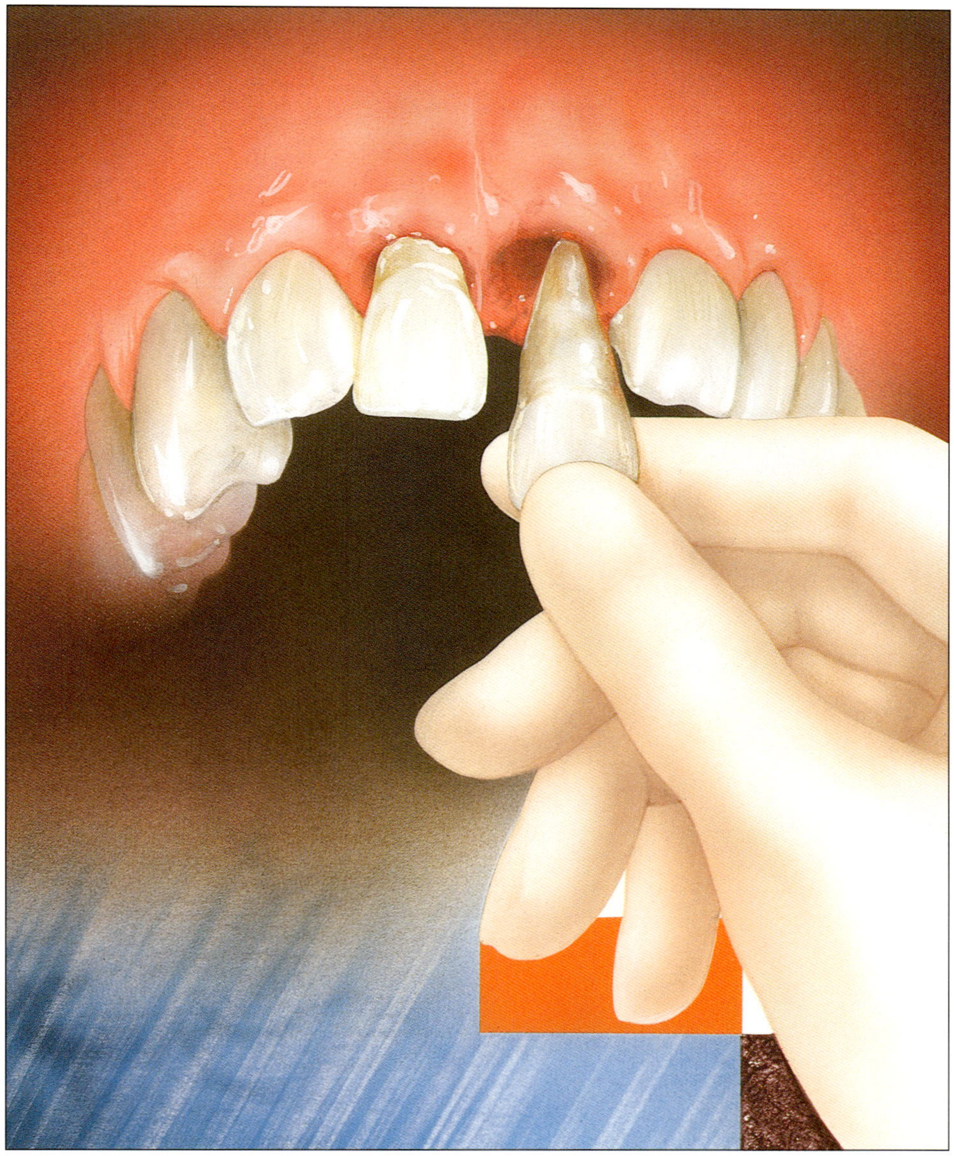

Replantation of avulsed teeth can be divided into two categories: those that are replanted within a short time (or preserved in a storage medium) and those that are replanted after a delay during which the periodontal membrane attached to the root has dried. In this chapter, consideration is also given to wound healing that involves both pulp and periodontal ligament tissue.

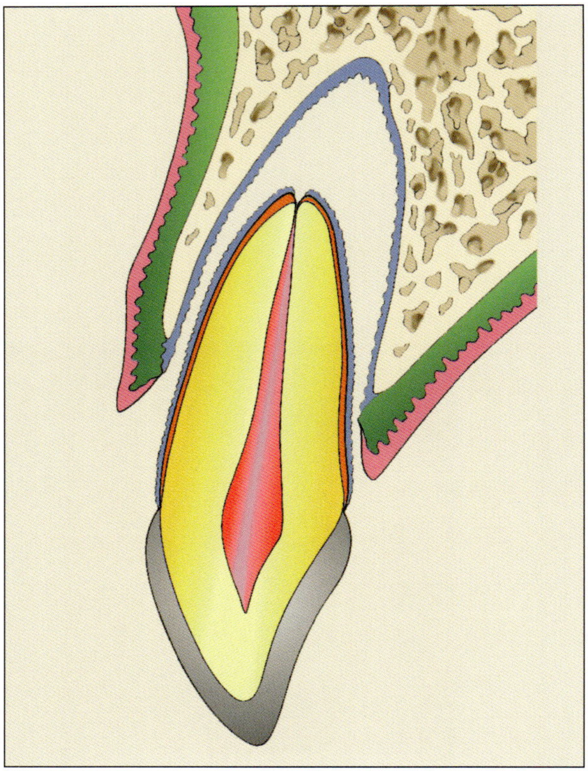

Fig 9-1 Avulsion.

Description

In avulsion, the entire tooth is completely separated from the supporting tissue (the alveolus and gingiva) (Fig 9-1).

Examination and Diagnosis: Key Points

An avulsed tooth can usually be retained by replantation; however, the prognosis depends on the extra-alveolar duration, the condition of the avulsed tooth, the patient's age, and root development.

In avulsion, the periodontal membrane is separated; half is attached to the root and the other half to the alveolus. Vitality of the periodontal membrane attached to the root is of great importance to the success of a replanted tooth. Exposed to air, the periodontal ligament (PDL) dries and becomes necrotic; after 30 minutes of dryness, the odds of recovery are significantly reduced.

Endodontic treatment should be delayed in an immature tooth because the pulp may revascularize after replantation. It is also important to recognize that replanting a tooth with a necrotic pulp causes inflammatory root resorption; therefore, careful postoperative observation is necessary. In the case of delayed replantation, there is a definite difference in results depending on the patient's age. In children, delayed replantation is usually not successful long term, making it important to discuss options thoroughly with the child's parents.

Treatment Plan

Replantation should be attempted whenever possible. However, the healing mechanisms of immediate replantation and delayed replantation are different. In immediate replantation, the replantation is given priority over endodontic treatment. In delayed replantation, endodontic treatment is performed outside the oral cavity with a calcium hydroxide preparation before the tooth is replanted. In delayed replantation, the periodontal membrane is considered necrotic.

Treatment Procedures

Immediate replantation

Immediate replantation is performed when the periodontal membrane of an avulsed tooth is considered vital. Replantation within 45 minutes of avulsion is considered immediate replantation. If the tooth is preserved in milk or in a preservative solution and is replanted within 24 hours, that is also considered immediate replantation.

1. *Preservation of the avulsed tooth*: When a patient calls to report an avulsion, give clear instructions about what to do with the tooth. It may be preserved in milk, in the mouth (Figs 9-2d and e), or in a commercial preservative solution (see Fig 9-17). During the office visit, preserve the avulsed tooth in a physiologic saline solution (Fig 9-2f).
2. *Examination and diagnosis*: Inspect the tooth and mouth, obtain the history, and perform a radiographic examination to determine the condition of the surrounding alveolus (Figs 9-2a to c).
3. *Cleansing of the avulsed tooth*: If it is difficult to remove contaminants from the periodontal membrane, use an ultrasonic cleaner with physiologic saline solution for 3 minutes. Be sure to wrap the tooth with gauze. For a severely contaminated tooth, use the ultrasonic scaler for debridement of the root surface while irrigating with physiologic saline solution, removing only the contaminant (within 30 seconds) (Fig 9-2g).
4. *Cleansing of the alveolus*: Irrigate blood clots from the alveolar socket.
5. *Replantation and splinting*: Place the avulsed tooth gently into the socket and splint it. If the adaptation between the replanted tooth and gingiva is poor, suture the gingiva to achieve close adaptation of the gingiva and cervical region. Use an orthodontic twisted wire (3M Unitek) and conventional adhesive resin for splinting (Figs 9-2h and i). Avoid splinting too tightly; persistent pressure to the replanted tooth may affect the outcome.
6. *Endodontic treatment*: In a mature tooth, endodontic treatment begins before splint removal (1 to 2 weeks after replantation). Use a calcium hydroxide preparation (Vitapex, Neo) for the initial filling and monitor the periodontal healing (Fig 9-2j). In an immature tooth, wait until pulp necrosis can be confirmed, because pulp tissue may revascularize. If inflammatory root resorption is noted, begin endodontic treatment immediately.
7. *Splint removal and follow-up*: Remove the splint after 2 to 3 weeks (Fig 9-2k). Examine carefully for any root resorption and pulp necrosis (Figs 9-2l to n).
8. *Final root canal filling*: Following the initial treatment of an avulsed tooth with necrotic pulp, use sealer and gutta-percha points for final root canal filling after confirming apical closure (Fig 9-2o).
9. *Bleaching and restorative treatment*: Bleach the tooth if necessary (see Chapter 6). Discoloration is common in nonvital teeth. Use composite resin to fill the lingual access. Continue to monitor the tooth (Figs 9-2p to r).

Fig 9-2 Immediate replantation

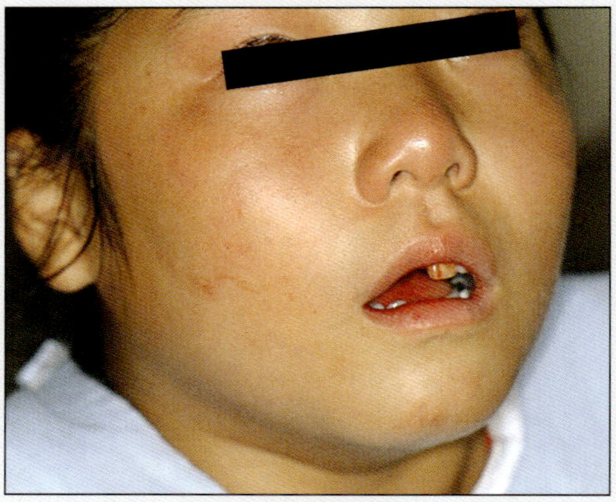
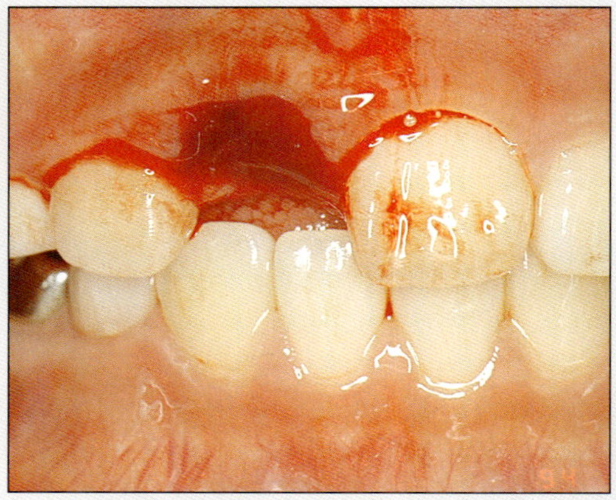
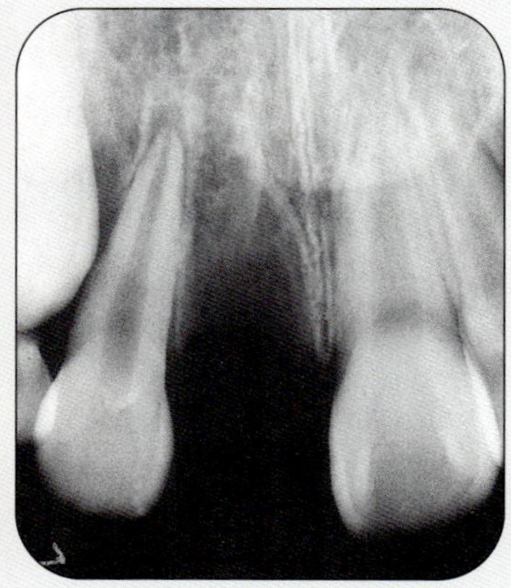

Figs 9-2a to c Preoperative view, 10-year-old girl. The initial visit is 15 minutes after the avulsion of tooth 8.

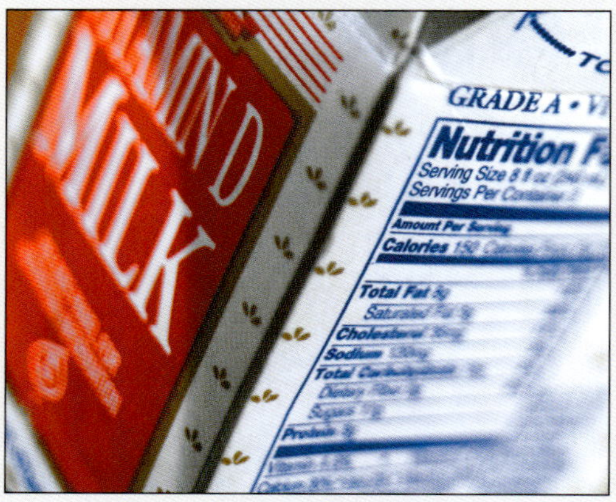

Fig 9-2d An avulsed tooth can be preserved in milk.

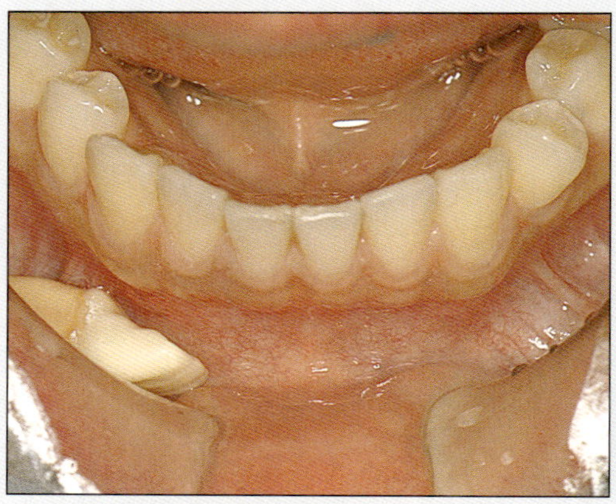

Fig 9-2e An avulsed tooth can be kept in the vestibule of the oral cavity.

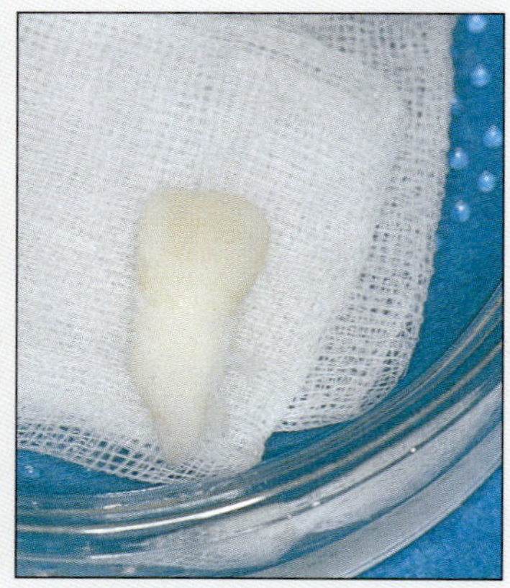

Fig 9-2f An avulsed tooth can be stored in physiologic saline solution.

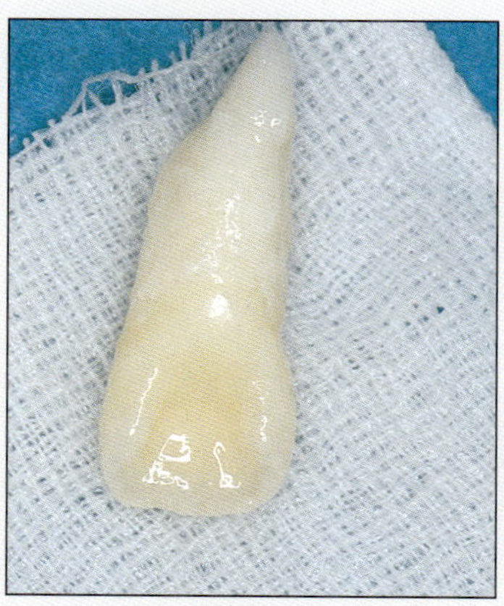

Fig 9-2g Cleansing of the avulsed tooth.

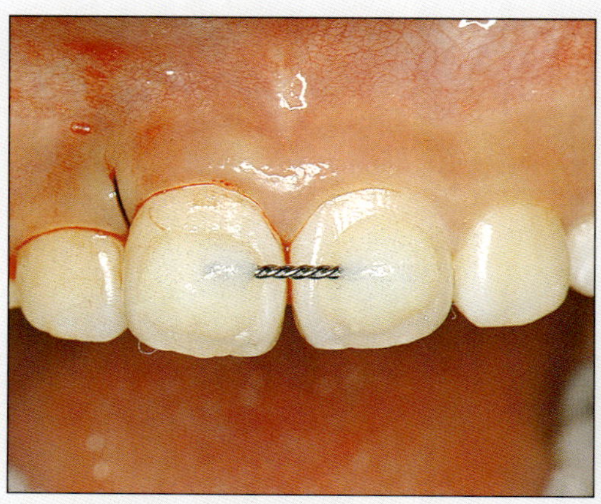

Fig 9-2h After replantation, suturing, and splinting.

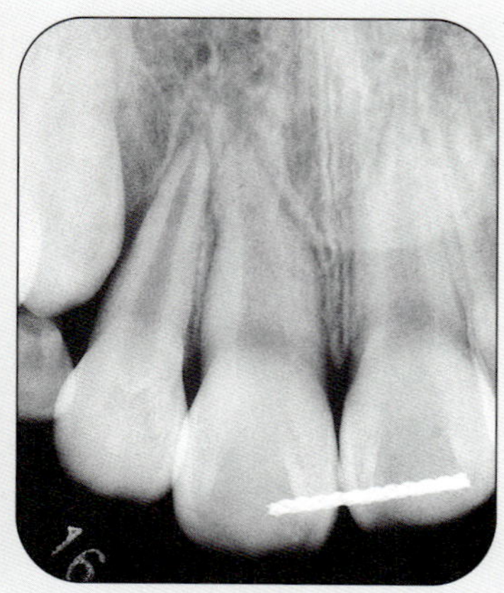

Fig 9-2i Radiographic confirmation.

Fig 9-2 (Continued)

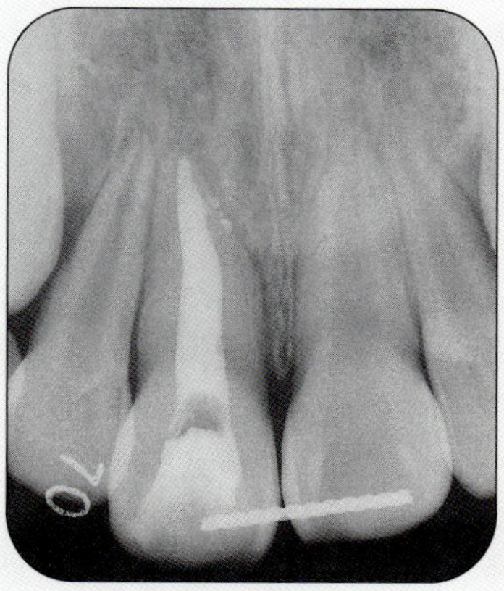

Fig 9-2j Two weeks after replantation, calcium hydroxide is placed in the root canal.

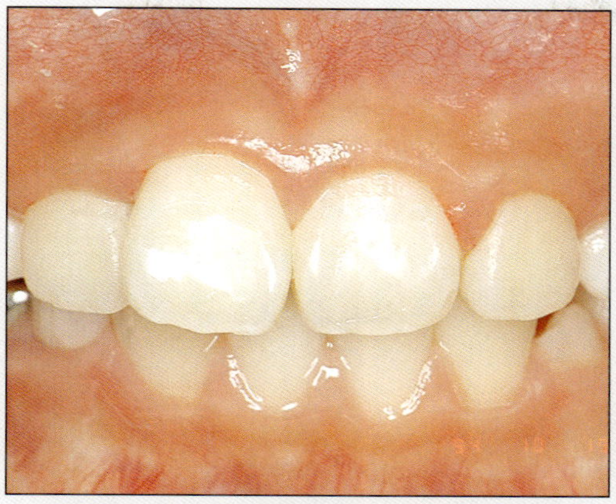

Fig 9-2k The splint is removed about 3 weeks after placement.

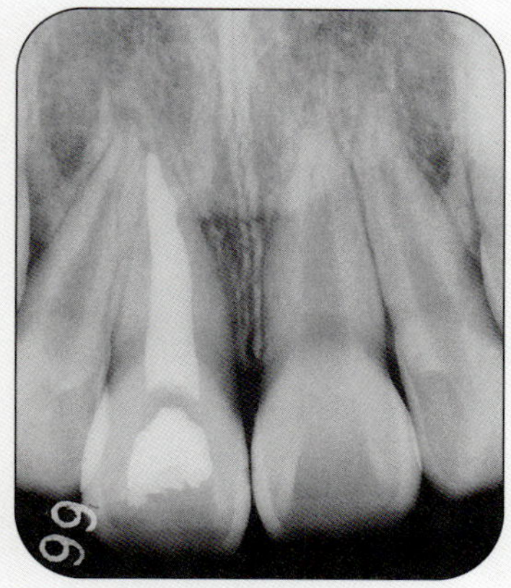

Fig 9-2l Six months later.

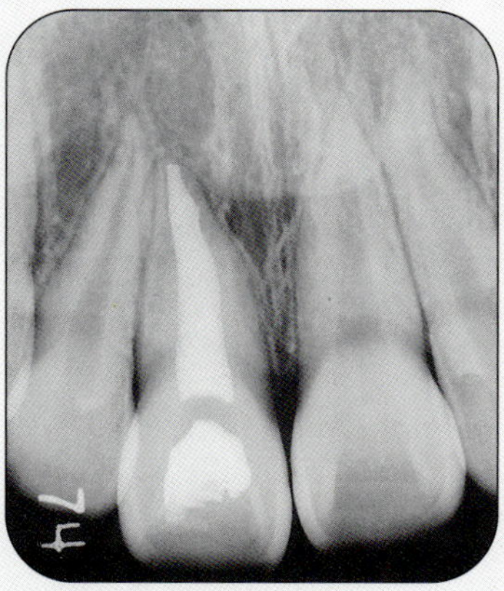

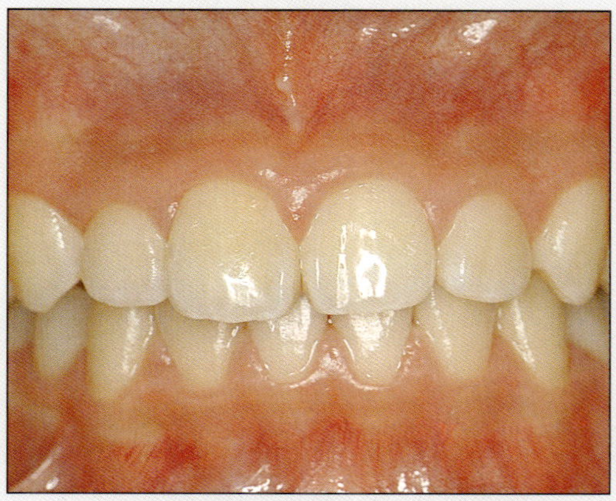

Figs 9-2m and n One year later.

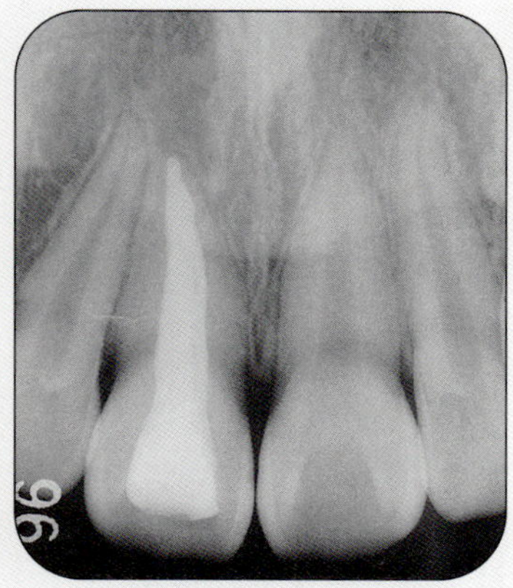

Fig 9-2o Three years later.

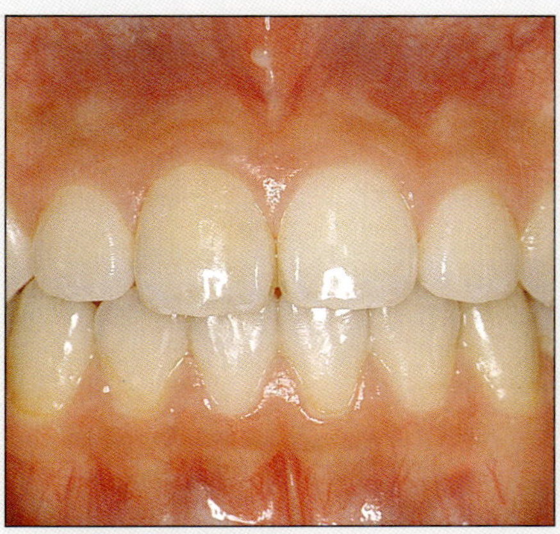

Fig 9-2p Three years later, before bleaching of the replanted tooth.

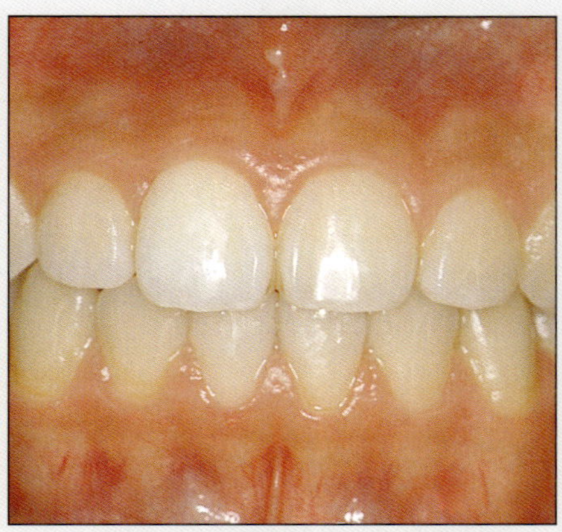

Fig 9-2q After bleaching and restorative treatment.

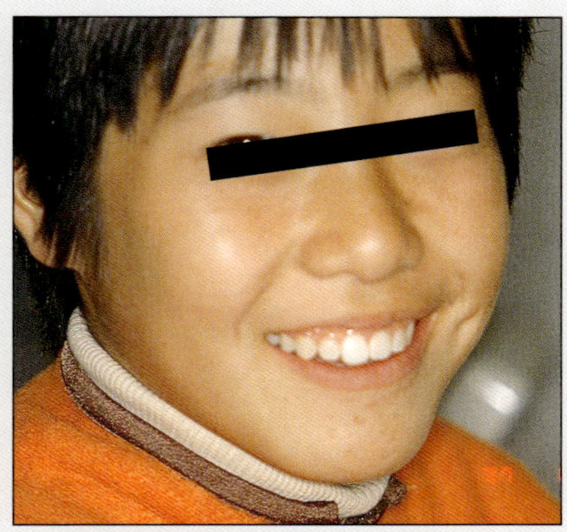

Fig 9-2r Facial view after bleaching and restorative treatment.

Fig 9-3 Delayed replantation in the adult patient

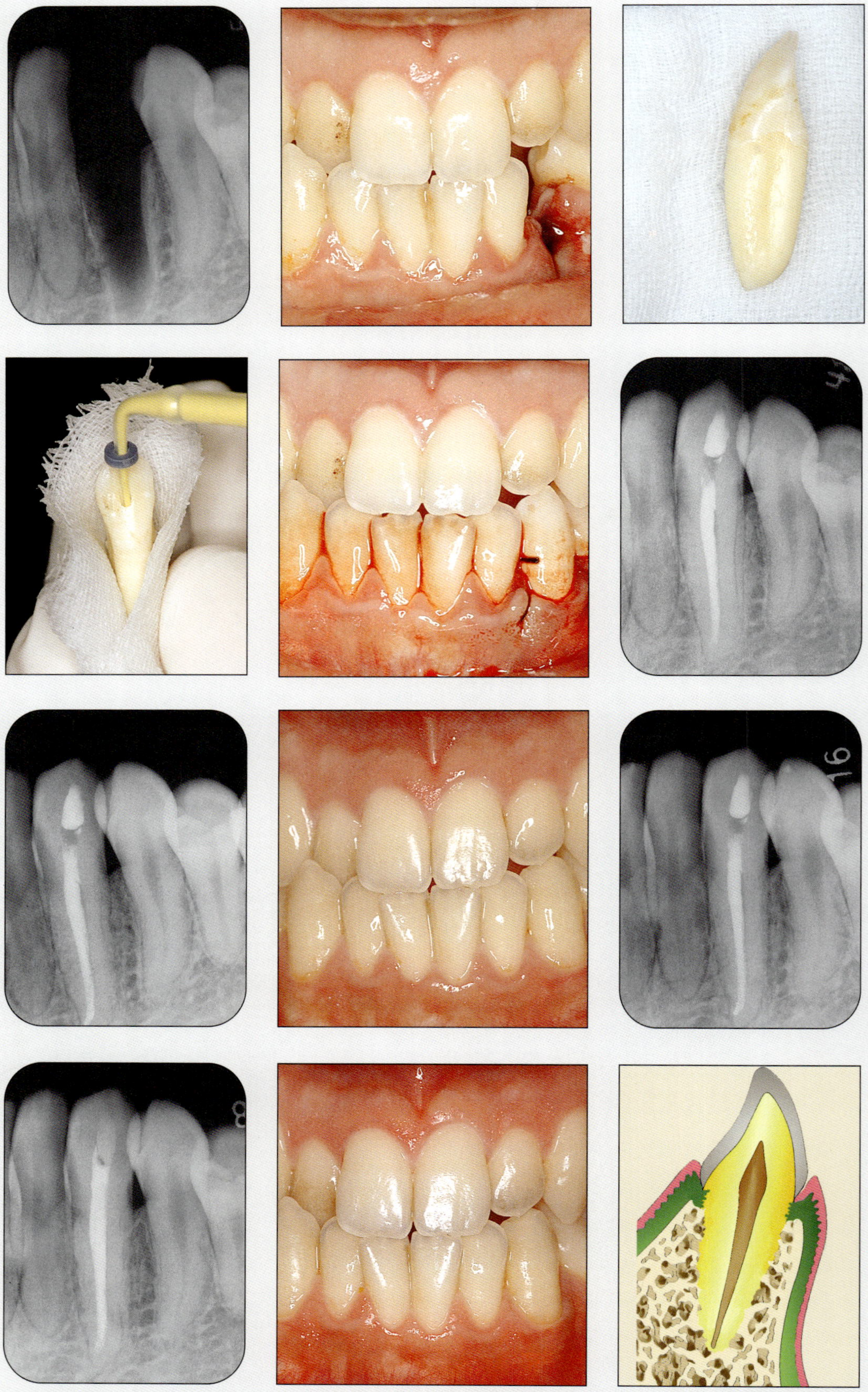

Figs 9-3a and b Preoperative views, 18-year-old man. The initial visit is 14 hours after avulsion.

Fig 9-3c Debriding and cleansing of the tooth. The attached periodontal ligament is not removed.

Fig 9-3d Root canal treatment extraorally. A calcium hydroxide preparation is used for the initial root canal filling.

Fig 9-3e Replantation and suture. While splinting is usually necessary, in this case, it is not because of good adaptation.

Fig 9-3f Immediately after replantation.

Fig 9-3g Six months later.

Figs 9-3h and i One year later.

Figs 9-3j and k Two years later. Ankylosis of the root is in progress, even though the clinical appearance is normal.

Fig 9-3l Ankylosis.

Fig 9-4 Delayed replantation, following initial healing of alveolar sockets (Courtesy of Dr Masanori Miyazaki)

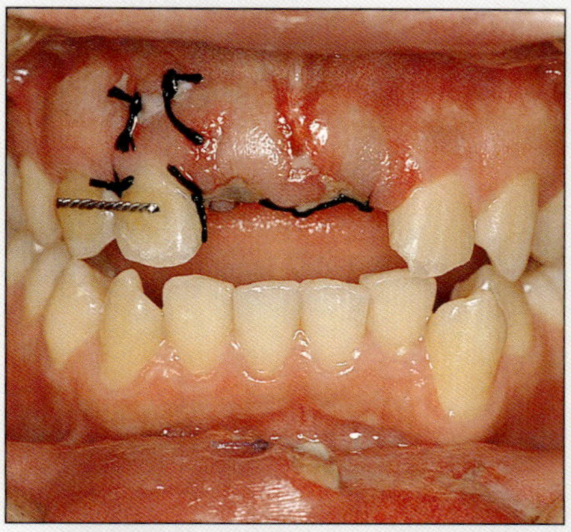

Fig 9-4a Preoperative view, 17-year-old boy. The initial visit is 2 days after trauma.

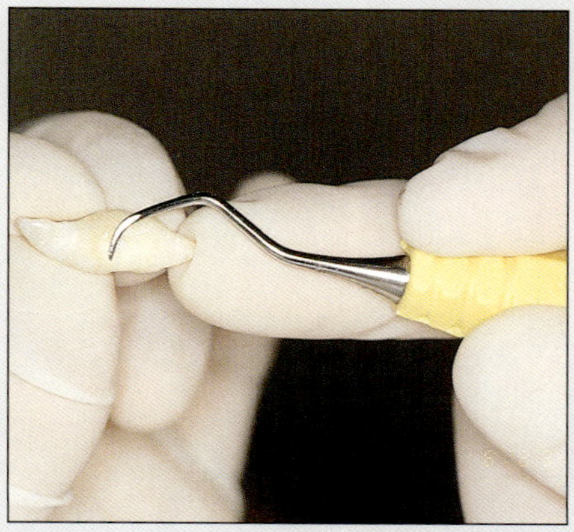

Fig 9-4b Removal of the periodontal ligament before replantation.

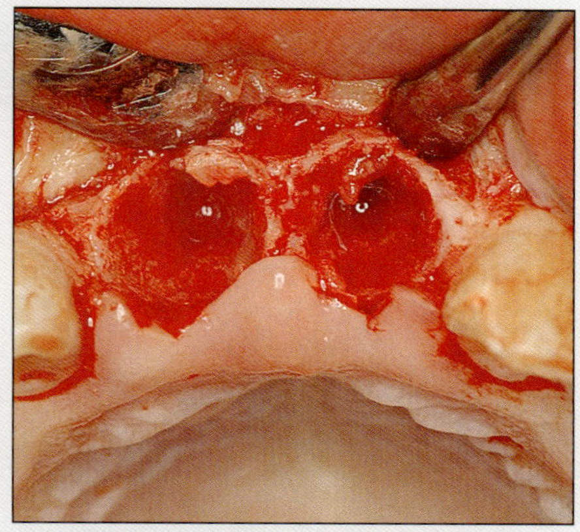

Fig 9-4c Preparation of the alveolar sockets because replantation occurred 17 days after trauma.

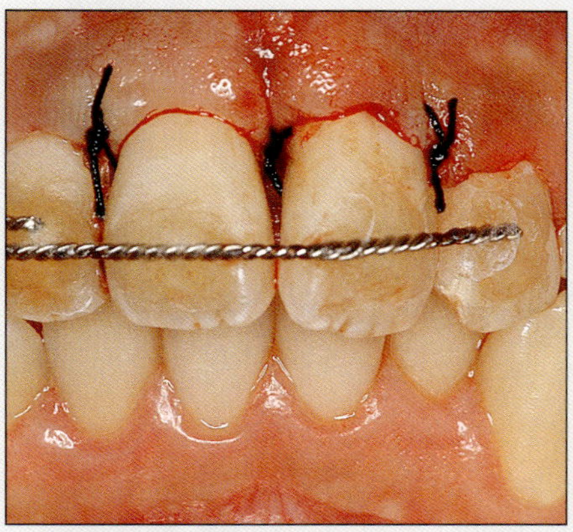

Fig 9-4d After replantation, suturing, and splinting.

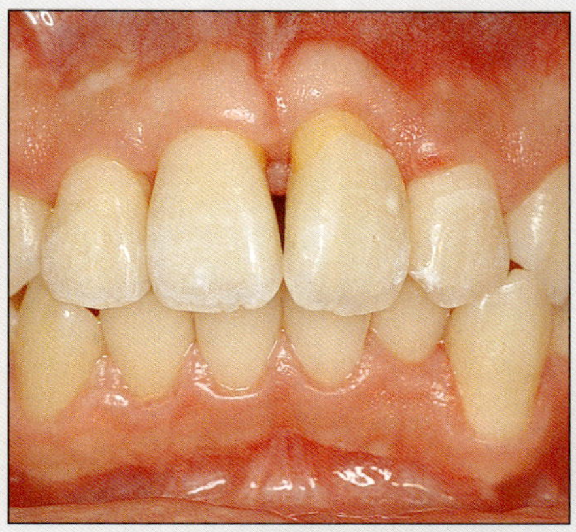

Fig 9-4e Two months later. The gingiva has receded noticeably.

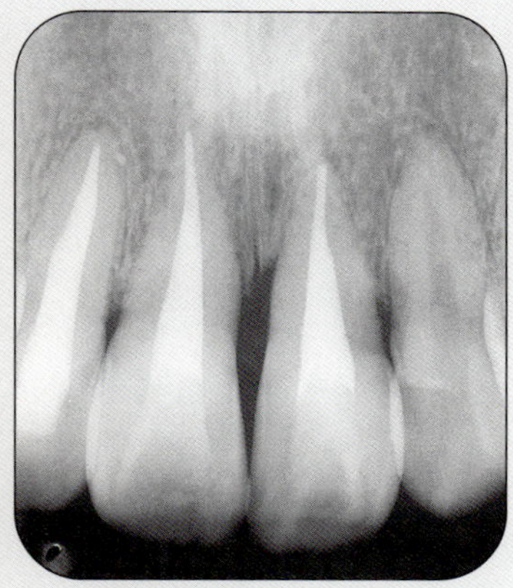

Fig 9-4f One year later. Note ankylosis involving the apexes of the replanted teeth.

Delayed replantation

Delayed replantation is the replanting of an avulsed tooth with a necrotic periodontal ligament. Even in delayed replantation, the tooth should be replanted at the initial visit if possible (Fig 9-3). The more advanced the healing of the alveolus, the more difficult replantation and desired healing becomes (Fig 9-4).

1. *Cleansing of the avulsed tooth*: Use ultrasonic cleansing with physiologic saline solution. If it is difficult to remove the contaminant, use an ultrasonic scaler. However, do not remove periodontal ligament fibers from the root surface (Fig 9-3c). Removing collagen fibers from the root surface by root planing may cause pocket formation and gingival recession after replantation. It may also reduce the longevity of the replanted tooth (Fig 9-4).
2. *Extraoral endodontic treatment*: In delayed replantation, perform endodontic treatment before replanting the tooth. Perform conventional enlargement and cleansing of the root canal and fill with a calcium hydroxide preparation (Fig 9-3d). Calcium hydroxide aids asepsis of the root canal.

Fig 9-5 Delayed replantation in the young patient

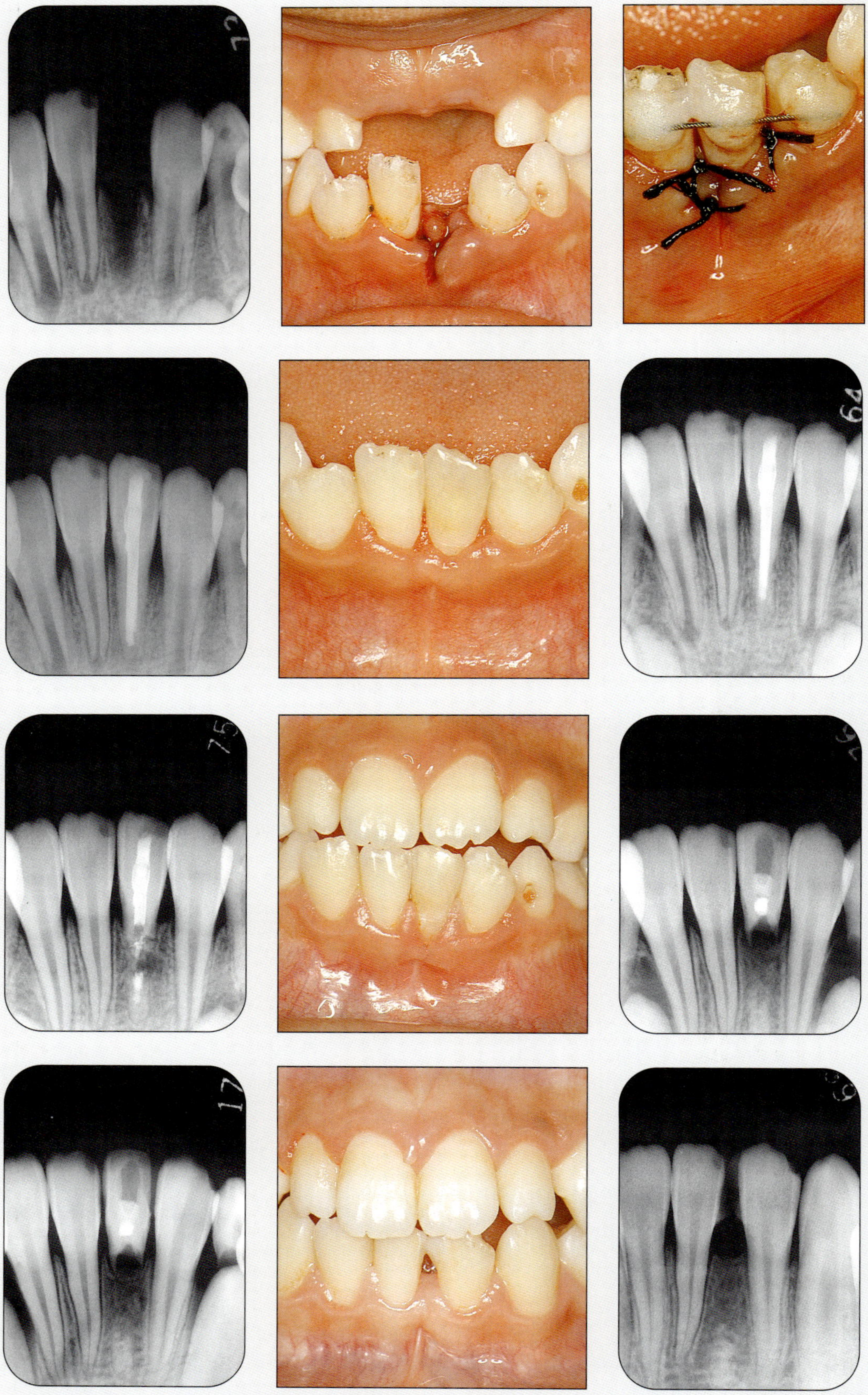

Figs 9-5a and b Preoperative views, 8-year-old boy. The initial visit is approximately 1 hour after trauma.

Fig 9-5c Immediately after replantation.

Figs 9-5d and e Two months later.

Fig 9-5f Six months later. Root resorption (ankylosis) is in progress.

Fig 9-5g One year later.

Figs 9-5h and i Two years later. Most of the root is resorbed.

Fig 9-5j Two years and 6 months later.

Figs 9-5k and l Five years later. The area is closing by natural exfoliation of the replanted tooth and tooth migration.

Fig 9-6 Delayed replantation and infraocclusion

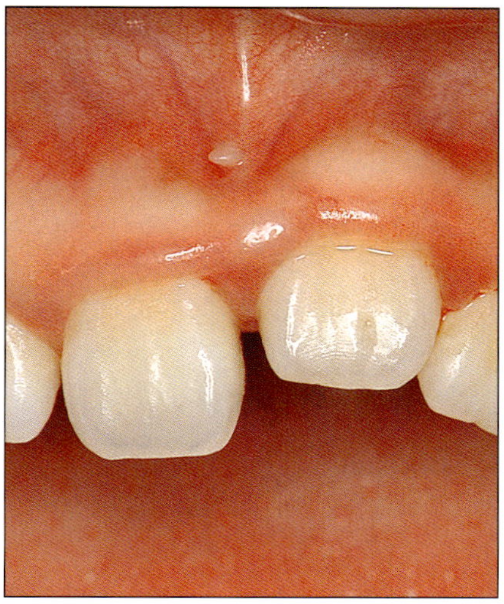

Fig 9-6a Infraocclusion due to ankylosis.

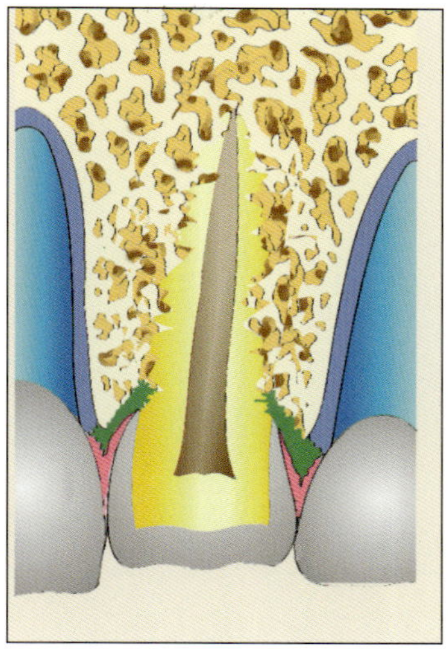

Fig 9-6b Ankylosis of a tooth replanted during puberty prevents its normal eruption. However, the healthy adjacent teeth continue to erupt; therefore, there is relative infraocclusion of the replanted tooth, which will eventually exfoliate.

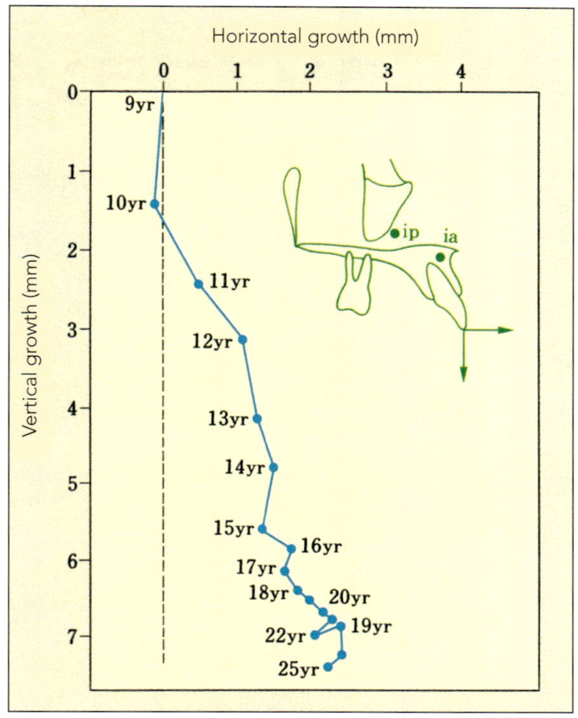

Fig 9-6c Tooth eruption and the amount of growth of alveolar bone.[94] It is possible to predict the degree of future infraocclusion by age when ankylosis of a replanted tooth occurs. For example, in a 12-year-old child, about 4 mm infraocclusion is likely when the patient reaches maturity. Reprinted from Andreasen and Andreasen.[7]

3. *Curettage and cleansing of the alveolar socket*: Perform curettage and irrigation to remove blood clots and granulation tissue from the socket.
4. *Replantation and splinting*: Replant and splint the tooth (Figs 9-3e and f).
5. *Removal of splint*: Remove the splint after about 4 weeks.
6. *Complete endodontic treatment*: In a mature tooth, replace the calcium hydroxide preparation with sealer and gutta-percha. In an immature root, leave the calcium hydroxide preparation or fill the canal with calcium hydroxide again, if necessary.
7. *Prognosis*: The goal of delayed replantation is ankylosis (Fig 9-3l); therefore, it is important to understand the rate at which root resorption occurs (Figs 9-3g to k). The speed of root resorption due to ankylosis differs prepuberty and postpuberty. In prepuberty patients (during growth and development), the root will be resorbed in approximately 2 years (Fig 9-5). In postpuberty patients (after growth and development), root resorption may take more than 10 years (Fig 9-3). If ankylosis occurs in pubescent patients (when growth and development gradually cease), unesthetic conditions and poor function will result. This is called infraocclusion (Fig 9-6). In such cases, the coronal part of the replanted tooth should be removed to the level of the cervical line.
8. *Treatment of resorbed replanted tooth*: When a replanted tooth is lost due to root resorption, choose a treatment such as autotransplantation of another tooth if one is available, an implant, or movement of teeth orthodontically to recover esthetics and function. The choice of treatment requires careful patient evaluation.

Fig 9-7 Reattachment after replantation

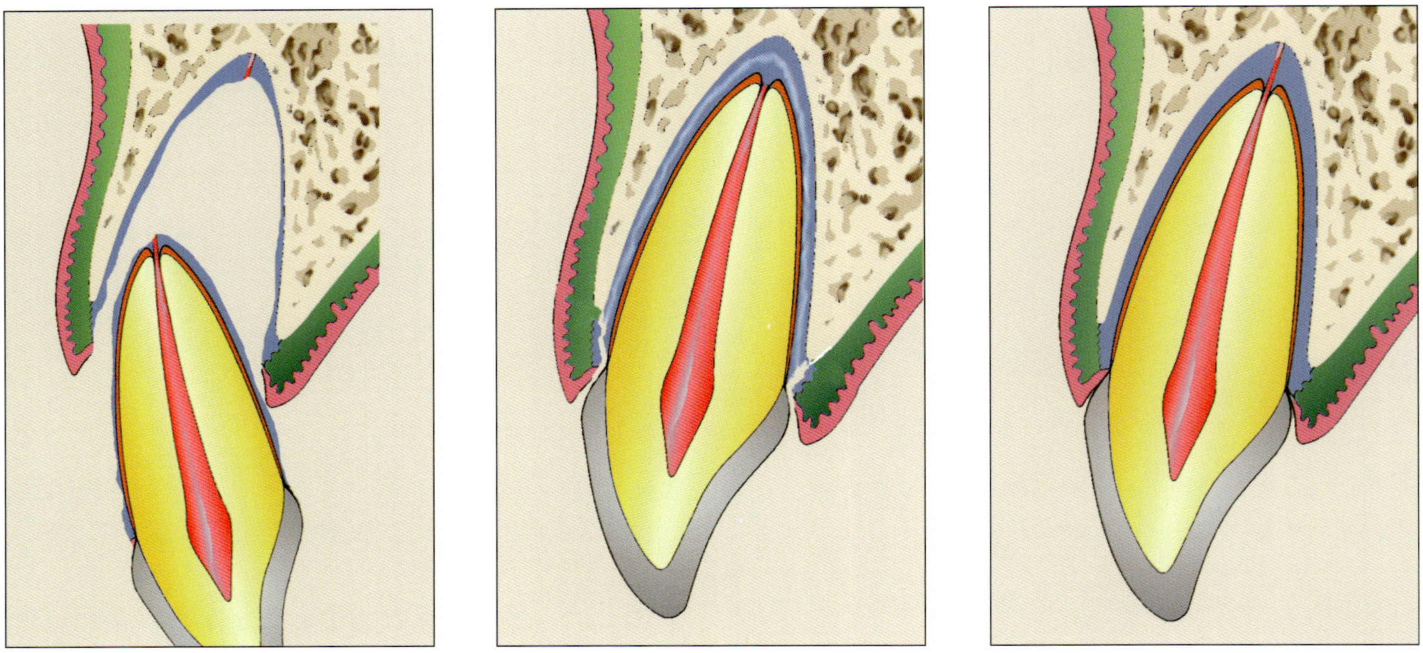

Fig 9-7a Before replantation. There is periodontal membrane both in the alveolus and on the avulsed tooth.

Fig 9-7b Immediately after replantation. Reattachment of periodontal fibers occurs between the fibers of the periodontal membrane attached to the root surface and those from the gingival connective tissue and alveolar socket.

Fig 9-7c After healing.

Wound Healing in Replantation

Healing of the periodontal membrane (reattachment and new attachment)

Healing of the periodontal membrane after replantation is by reattachment.[49-54] The ideal reattachment is the reorganization of connective tissue from the periodontal membrane attached to the root surface and gingival connective tissue or periodontal membrane tissue of the alveolus in a relatively short period of time (about 2 weeks). Usually, coronal to the alveolar bone margin, reattachment of the gingival connective tissue and periodontal membrane of the root occurs in 2 to 7 days. In the alveolus, reattachment occurs in 2 weeks[33] (Fig 9-7). If there is no healthy periodontal membrane on the replanted tooth, normal reattachment cannot occur.

In replantation of a tooth with a partially missing vital periodontal membrane, the healing of the membrane requires new attachment.[55-65] The new attachment develops from regeneration of periodontal membrane tissue with deposition of cementum (Fig 9-8). Therefore, most of the periodontal healing after replantation depends on reattachment and healing of partially missing periodontal membrane by new attachment. Extensive periodontal membrane damage or necrosis of a replanted tooth, however, results in root resorption.

Fig 9-8 New attachment

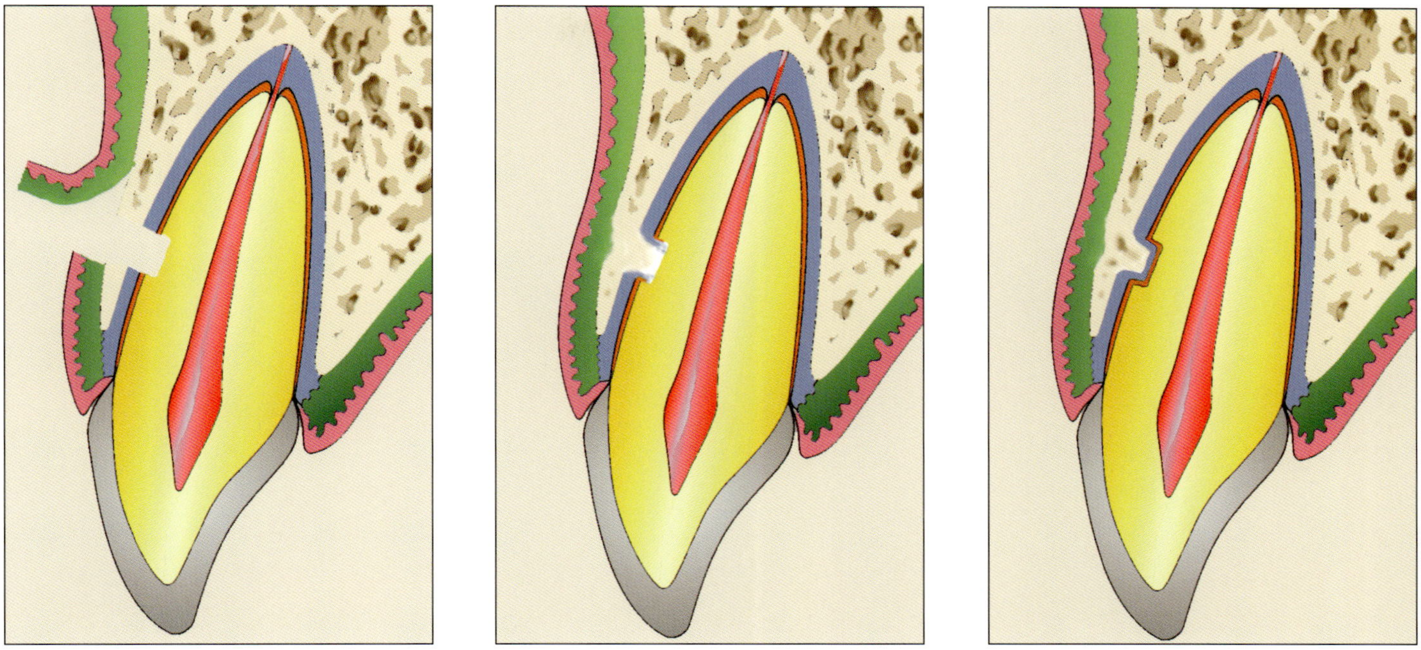

Fig 9-8a Experimental removal of periodontal tissue with a fenestration from the oral vestibule and removal of alveolar bone, periodontal membrane, and cementum to prepare a small cavity in the dentin.

Fig 9-8b During healing. Cells proliferate from the surrounding periodontal membrane and invade the cavity in the dentin.

Fig 9-8c After healing. The periodontal membrane tissue regenerates while depositing cementum in the cavity. The bone tissue regenerates from the periphery. There is new attachment between the periodontal membrane and the bone tissue.

Pulpal treatment and root development

In an immature tooth, pulpal healing[44,46,47,66] and root growth[67–71] can be expected after replantation. Pulp tissue becomes ischemic after tooth avulsion (Fig 9-9a). However, in case of a wide apex (more than 1 mm), it is possible for blood vessels to proliferate into the pulp cavity after replantation.[66,71] Blood vessels and pulp cells near the apex (inside Hertwig's epithelial sheath) proliferate coronally (Fig 9-9b). This proliferation proceeds at about 0.5 mm a day,[7] and the pulp cavity will be filled with vital tissue a few months after replantation. However, this regenerated pulp tissue rarely functions as before, and pulp canal obliteration occurs due to rapid deposition of hard tissue (osteodentin)[72–78] (Figs 9-9c and 9-10). The pulp may respond positively to the electric pulp test immediately after obliteration, but its future is uncertain.

Also, in cases where Hertwig's epithelial sheath (see Chapter 1) at the apex is vital, root growth can be expected after replantation (Fig 9-11). However, it is impossible to predict how much root there will be compared to normal development[67–71] (compare Figs 9-10 and 9-11).

Fig 9-9 Pulp healing

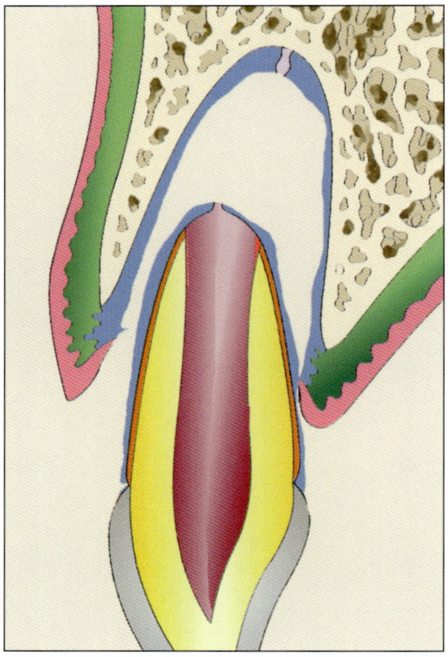

Fig 9-9a Avulsion of an immature tooth. The pulp changes ischemically.

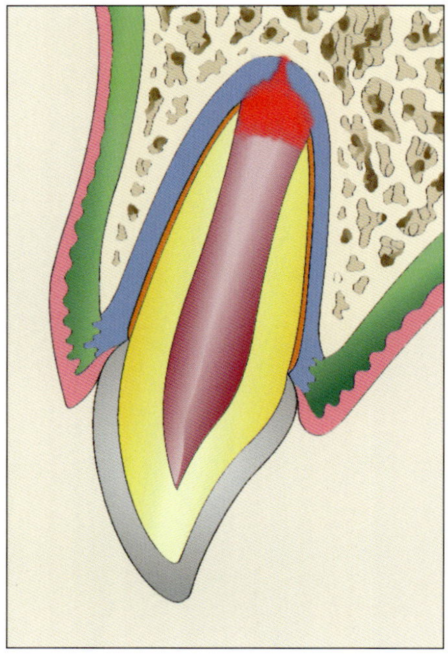

Fig 9-9b During healing. After replantation, blood capillaries proliferate and invade the pulp cavity from the apex, growing coronally.

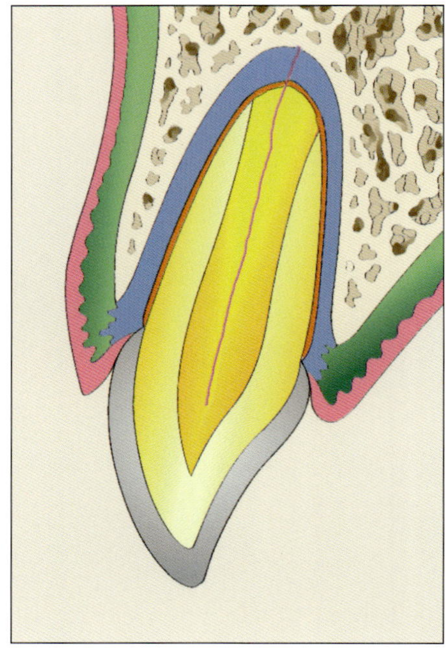

Fig 9-9c After healing. Proliferated pulp tissue in the pulp cavity calcifies rapidly, and the pulp cavity is obliterated.

Fig 9-10 Pulp obliteration after replantation

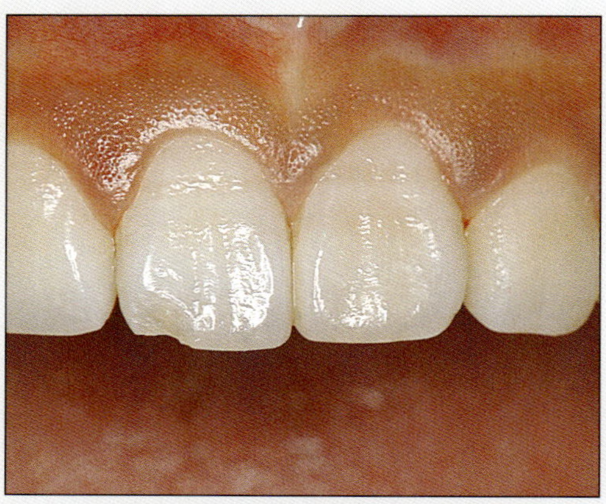

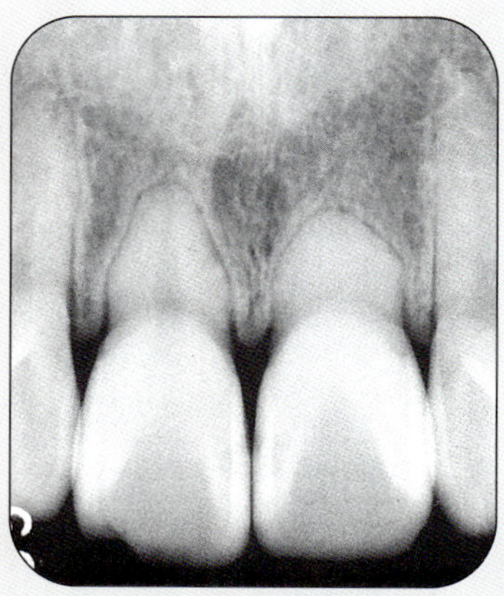

Figs 9-10a and b Twenty-two-year-old woman. Note the pulp obliteration of tooth 9, which was replanted about 13 years previously.

Phantom root and inner periodontal ligament

When there is trauma to the apical region of a developing root and Hertwig's epithelial root sheath is separated from the apex, a phantom root or inner PDL may develop (Fig 9-12).[7,79-83] Hertwig's epithelial root sheath cells, which originally formed the enamel epithelium, differentiate and reorganize to regenerate new tooth germs; therefore, a phantom root develops.

Fig 9-11 Continuous root development and pulp obliteration after intentional replantation

Fig 9-11a Radiograph immediately after replantation in a 10-year-old boy. Intentional replantation is performed to treat the delayed eruption of tooth 8.

Fig 9-11b One year and 6 months later. Note the root development and pulp obliteration.

Fig 9-11c Three years and 6 months later. Root development is nearly complete; however, pulp obliteration continues.

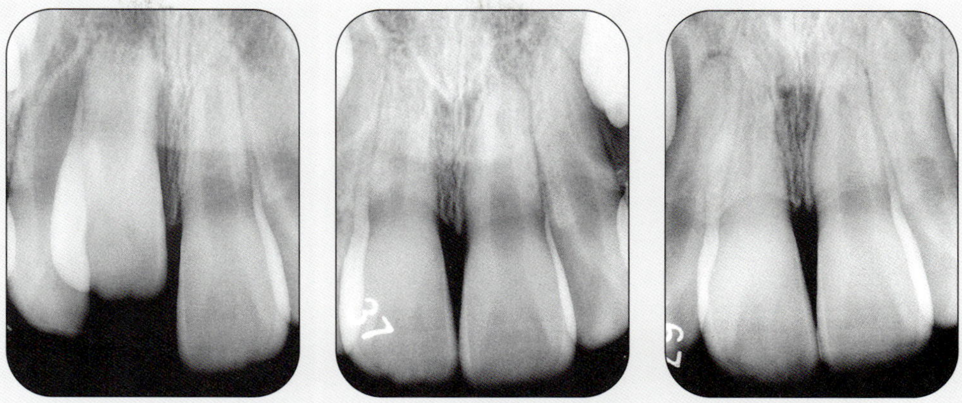

Fig 9-12 Formation of phantom root and inner periodontal ligament

(Courtesy of Dr Michiko Matsuura)

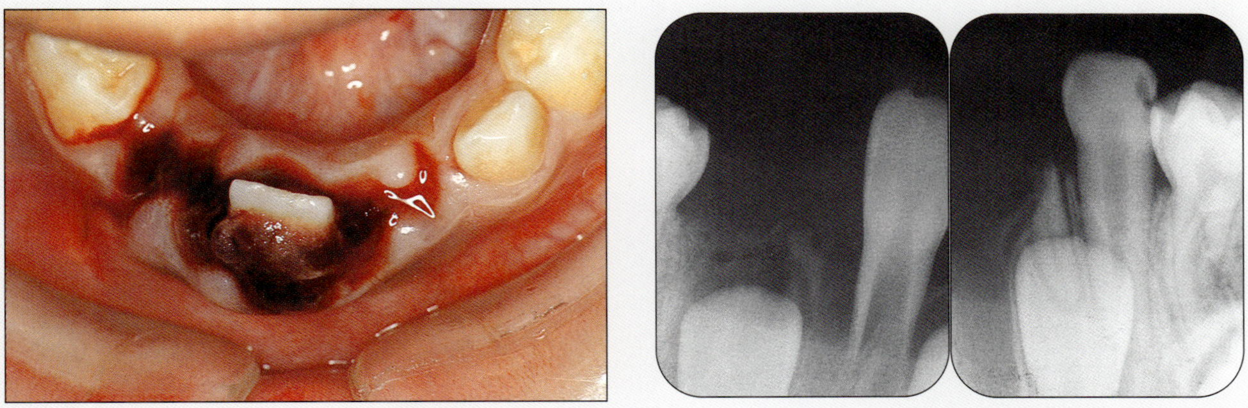

Figs 9-12a and b Preoperative view, 5-year-old boy with avulsed primary teeth N, Q, R and permanent tooth 24, and extrusively luxated tooth 25.

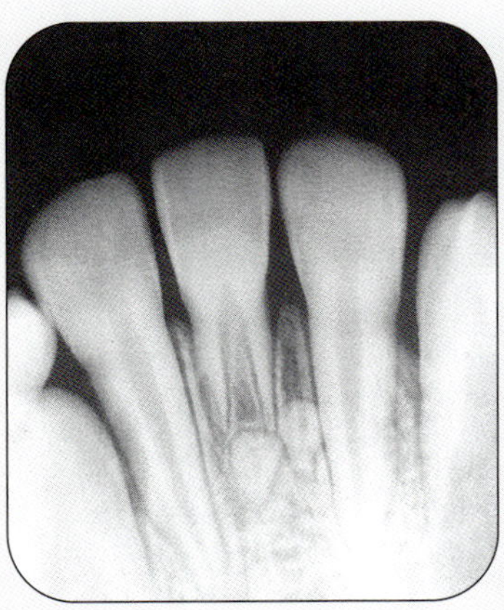

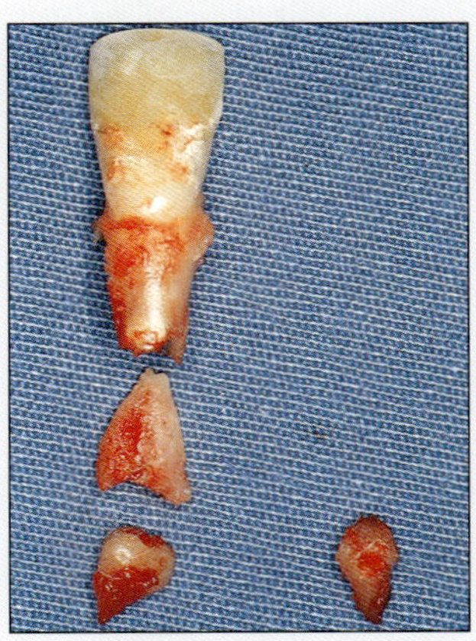

Fig 9-12c Three years later. Note the phantom roots in the apical area of tooth 25 and the avulsion site of tooth 24. In addition, the development of an inner PDL can be seen on the root of tooth 25.

Fig 9-12d Tooth 25, which was strategically extracted for orthodontic treatment, and two pieces of phantom roots. There is coronal formation on one phantom root thought to be enamel. During extraction, the area of inner PDL and the osseous tissue in the pulp cavity were removed.

Another outcome following replantation of immature teeth is the invasion of periodontal membrane tissue and osseous tissue into the pulp cavity (Fig 9-13), producing an inner PDL. The periodontal membrane tissue invades the pulp space apically and migrates coronally while depositing cementum. Osseous tissue also grows into the pulp space coronally.

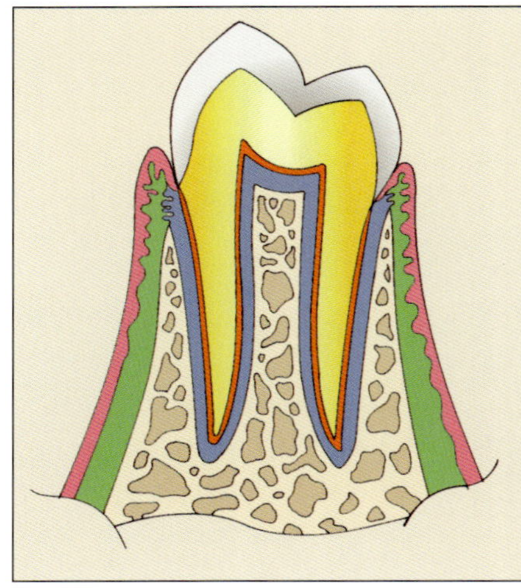

Fig 9-13 Inner periodontal ligament. The periodontal membrane from the root proliferates into the apical pulp cavity while depositing cementum. Simultaneously, osseous tissue proliferates into the pulp cavity.

Classification and mechanism of root resorption

If there is partial or complete necrosis of the periodontal membrane of a replanted tooth, root resorption occurs after replantation. Root resorption may be surface resorption, replacement resorption, or inflammatory resorption[84,85] (Fig 9-14). Currently, it is thought that osteoclasts participate in the resorption of hard tissue such as root or bone[86,87] and its mechanism continues to be elucidated[88] (Fig 9-15). Osteoclasts have two primary roles, physiologic remodeling of bone and defense of the body.[87] Following are explanations of the mechanism of each type of root resorption[89–92] and treatment.

Surface resorption. Surface resorption is limited to cementum, and repair occurs during the repair process of reattachment (see Fig 9-8). It is a generic term of a transient root resorption. Provided the stimulus for resorption (bacteria) is removed, the surface resorption will be repaired. If the bacterial stimulation is not removed, surface resorption will proceed to either replacement resorption or inflammatory resorption.

Replacement resorption. In this condition, which is also called ankylosis, bone and root are fused. This phenomenon can be seen both histologically and radiographically. The mechanism of replacement resorption of a tooth is remodeling with osseous tissue. In other words, it is caused by the coupling phenomenon where root resorption by osteoclasts lying in osseous tissue and bone deposition by osteoblasts occur simultaneously.[93] Therefore, the speed of replacement resorption correlates to the remodeling speed of bone (fast in young people and slow in adults). Approximately 50% of bone remodeling occurs in 1 year in children (prepuberty), while approximately 2% occurs in adults (postpuberty).[87] Age greatly affects the success rate of delayed replantation. Cases of ankylosis in children show that roots are resorbed within a few years (see Fig 9-5), a process that can take more than 10 years in adults (see Fig 9-3). Long-term esthetics and function, therefore, can be maintained in delayed replanted teeth in adults.

If ankylosis occurs after delayed replantation in pubescent patients (boys, 12 to 15 years; girls, 11 to 14 years), esthetics and function may be affected by infraocclusion (see Fig 9-6). Vertical growth of alveolar bone depends mainly on tooth eruption.[94] With ankylosis, the tooth will not erupt and the alveolar bone will not grow. The degree of infraocclusion is affected by the patient's age; the younger the age, the greater the degree of infraocclusion (see Fig 9-6c). In such cases, it is possible to recover normal alveolar height by reducing the ankylosed tooth crown to the level of the bone margin.

Fig 9-14 Classification of root resorption[85]

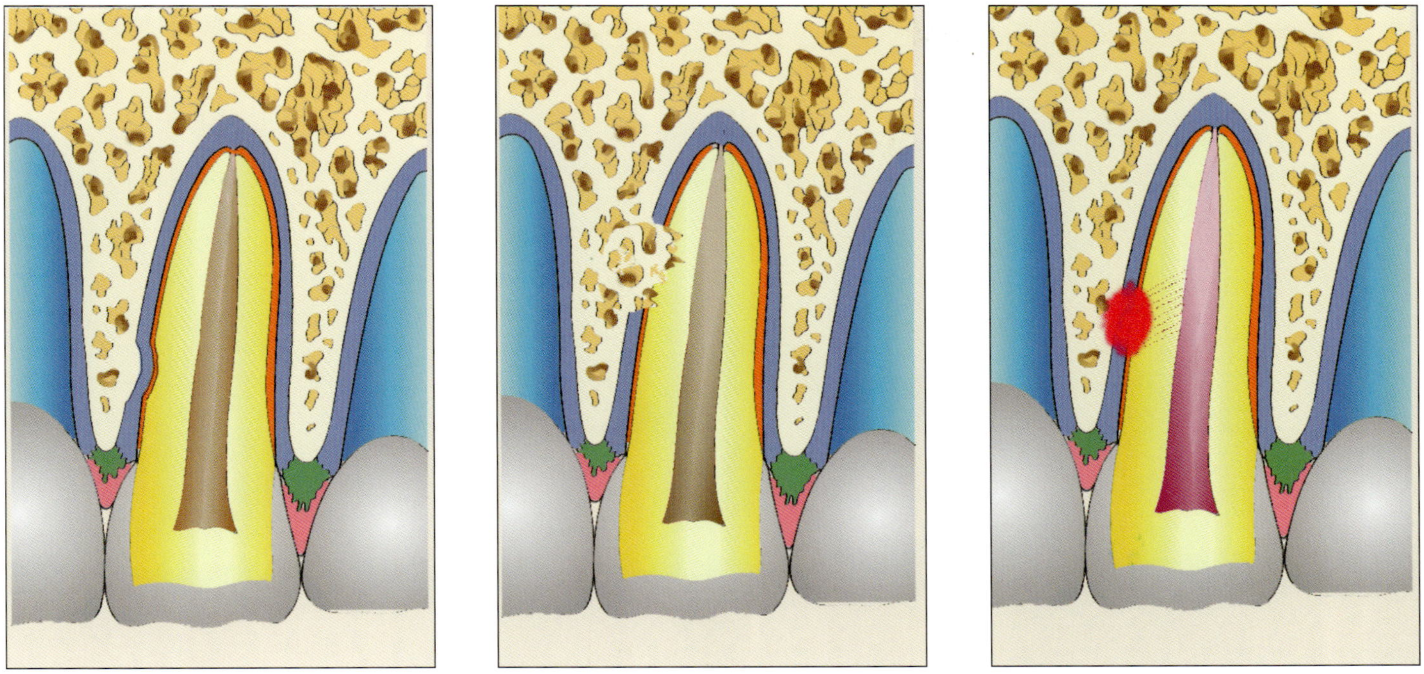

Fig 9-14a Surface resorption.

Fig 9-14b Replacement resorption.

Fig 9-14c Inflammatory resorption.

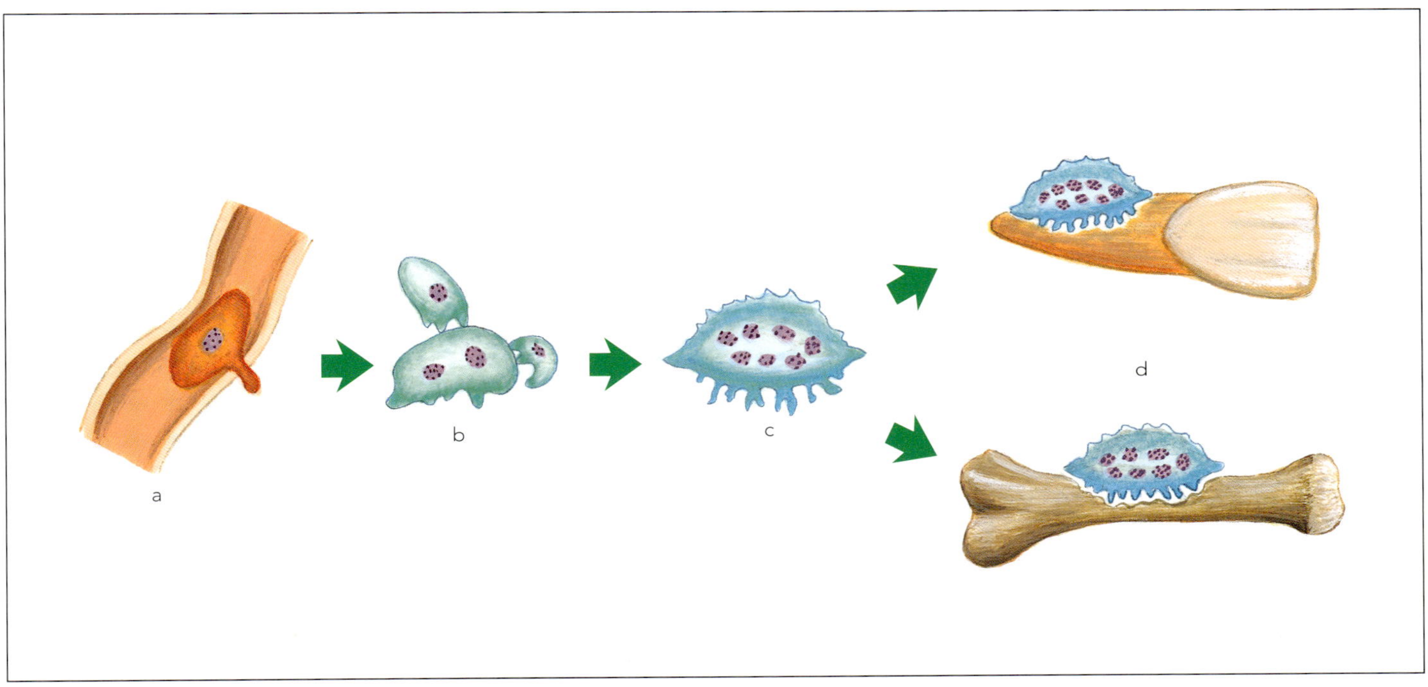

Fig 9-15 Developmental mechanism of the osteoclast.[88] Precursors in blood vessels migrate by chemotaxis of inflammatory transmitters (eg, interleukin) and hormones (a). Precursors fuse and differentiate (b) into mature, multinucleated osteoclasts (c). Osteoclasts participate in the resorption of hard tissue such as bone, cementum, and dentin (d).

Fig 9-16 Management of inflammatory resorption

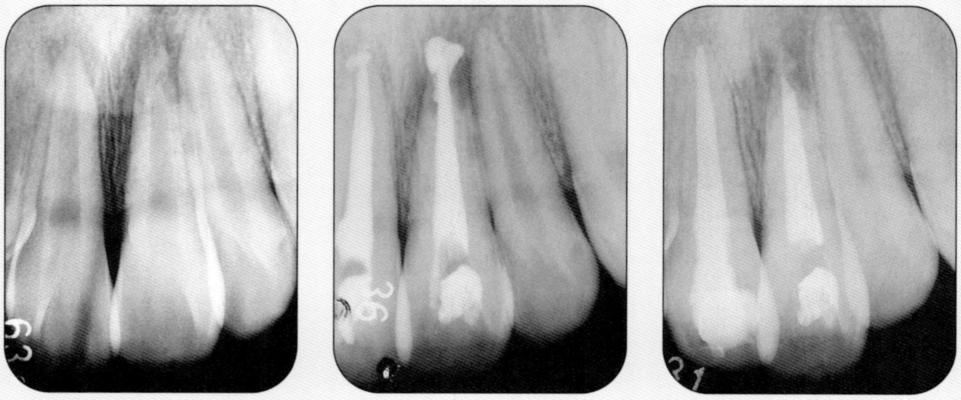

Fig 9-16a

Fig 9-16b

Fig 9-16c

Fig 9-16a Radiograph of 11-year, 10-month-old boy with subluxation of tooth 8 and avulsion of tooth 9, 2 months after replantation. Treatment was provided 30 minutes after trauma in another dental office. Note the inflammatory resorption of tooth 9.

Fig 9-16b After preparation of the canals of teeth 8 and 9. The pulps were necrotic. The initial root canal filling was calcium hydroxide.

Fig 9-16c Two years later. The inflammatory resorption of tooth 9 was arrested.

Inflammatory resorption. In a tooth with pulp necrosis, when cementum is resorbed by osteoclasts in an area of missing or necrotic periodontal membrane, dentinal tubules are exposed.[95,96] Necrotic material and bacteria from the pulp cavity reach the root surface through the exposed dentinal tubules, and an inflammatory response occurs. Root resorption is advanced by osteoclasts which emerge as the inflammatory process spreads[88] (Fig 9-15). Histologically, granulation tissue is present in the root resorption area, and, radiographically, radiolucencies are observed.

The speed of inflammatory resorption is affected by the degree of infection; however, it is relatively fast regardless of age. Resorption continues until the cause of infection is removed, which can be accomplished by root canal treatment (Fig 9-16). Following root canal treatment, new attachment can be expected if periodontal membrane cells invade the resorption areas. The same condition as in surface resorption will result, and root resorption will be contained. However, in cases of large resorption areas where osseous tissue reaches the root surface, inflammatory resorption may shift to replacement resorption. In such cases, the entire root may be resorbed.

Methods for the preservation of the periodontal membrane in avulsed teeth

Studies show positive results using storage media for preserving periodontal membrane cells outside the oral cavity.[97] Periodontal membrane on the root surface can survive when it is left in a dry condition for up to 18 minutes, more than half die in 30 minutes, and most die in 120 minutes (Table 9-1). Most periodontal membrane cells live for 120 minutes in physiologic saline solution; however, they will die before 120 minutes in water (Table 9-2).

Table 9-1 Survival rate of periodontal membrane in a dry condition[97]

Drying time (min)	Survival rate of periodontal membrane (%)
18	70.5 ± 17.3
30	28.2 ± 18.9
60	21.2 ± 13.4
90	15.2 ± 6.2
120	20.1 ± 19.7

Table 9-2 Survival rate of periodontal membrane in a moist condition[97]

Physiologic saline solution (min)	Survival rate of periodontal membrane (%)
18	80.0 ± 13.0
30	71.3 ± 18.2
60	71.4 ± 14.2
120	61.7 ± 11.4
Tap water (min)	
120	33.2 ± 12.2

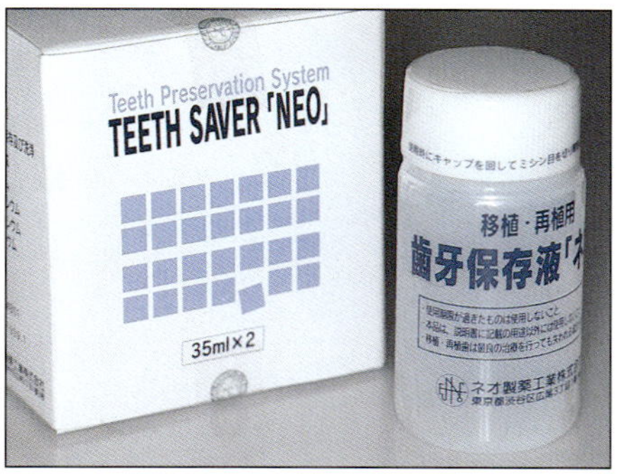

Fig 9-17 Preservative solution for transplantation or replantation of teeth. (It is available in the US as Save•A•Tooth, Smart Practice, Phoenix, AZ.) Soaking an avulsed tooth in this solution immediately after avulsion keeps the periodontal membrane vital for up to 24 hours.

Milk has long been known as a good preservative for avulsed teeth.[98,99] Ankylosis will not occur up to 6 hours after replantation if the avulsed tooth is preserved in milk.[99] There are also new preservative solutions for avulsed teeth and for use during tooth transplantation (Fig 9-17). The use of these solutions allows the periodontal membranes of avulsed teeth to survive up to 24 hours.[100,101]

Clinically, no more than 45 minutes should elapse between trauma and replantation if ankylosis is to be prevented. If the avulsed tooth remains in the oral cavity, it is preserved because of the moist condition. The periodontal membrane can live for a few hours, and the possibility of successful replantation increases.

10

Trauma to Supporting Structures

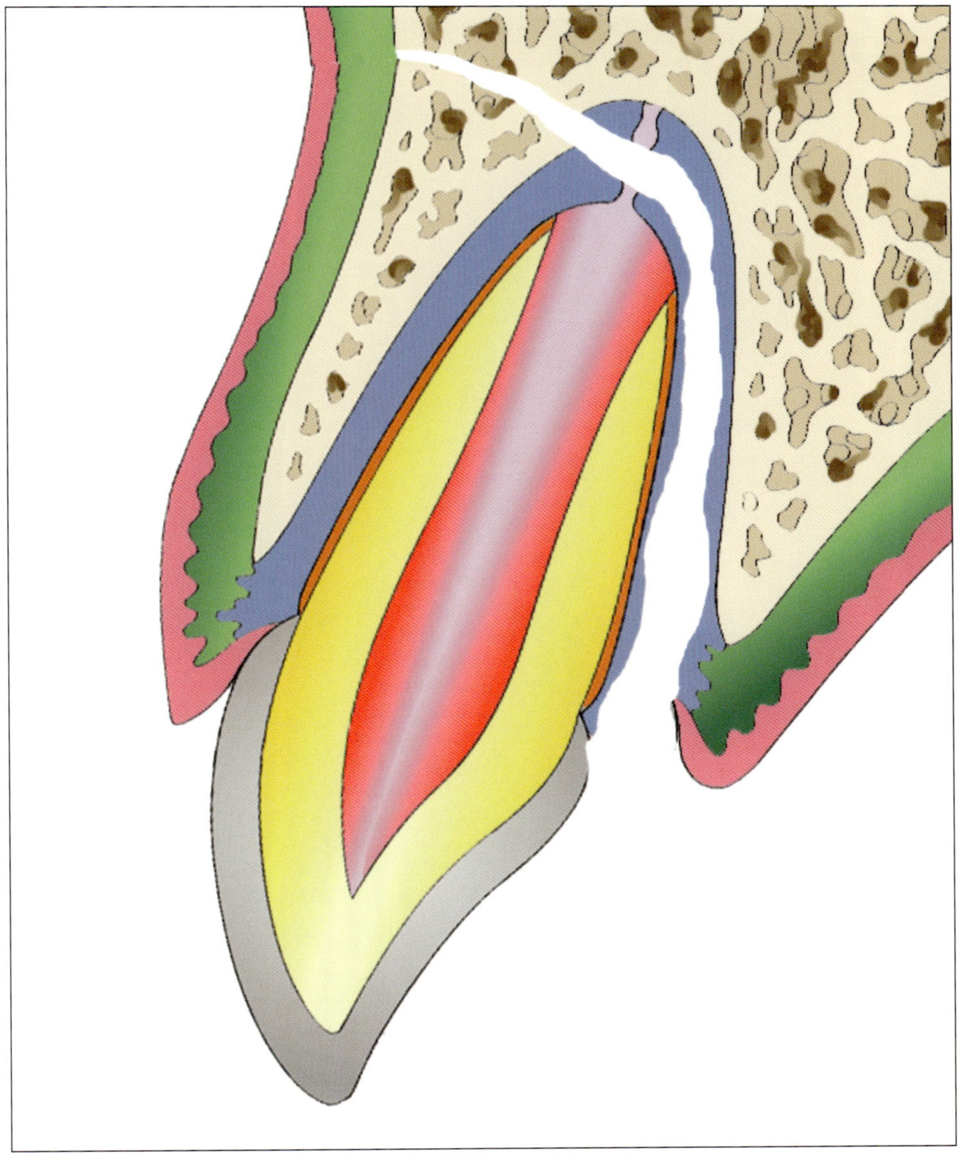

Injuries to teeth may be combined with fractures of the alveolar bone and the maxilla and mandible as well as soft tissue trauma to the gingiva and oral mucosa.

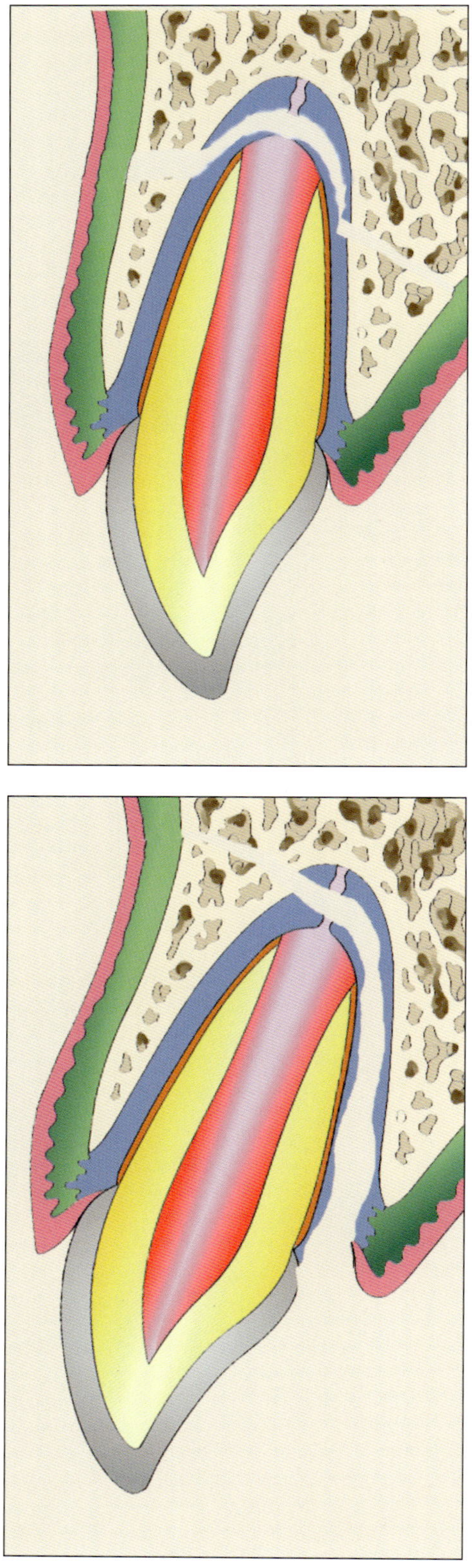

Figs 10-1a and b Alveolar bone fractures.

Trauma to the Maxilla or Mandible: Description

Alveolar bone fracture

This fracture involves the alveolar bone coronal to the apex. Usually the fracture line passes through the alveolus (Fig 10-1).

Fracture of maxilla and mandible

This is an extensive fracture of the basal bone and mandibular ramus. Usually the alveolar bone is also involved (Figs 10-2 and 10-3).

Examination and Diagnosis: Key Points

In cases of trauma involving multiple teeth, there may be complications such as alveolar bone fractures (Fig 10-4). Also, in cases of intrusive luxation and lateral luxation, there are usually also alveolar bone fractures. Careful examination of the radiographs for fractures is required.

In cases of posttrauma malocclusion, suspect fracture of the diaphysis even if there is no malposition of teeth (Fig 10-3). There are areas especially susceptible to fractures,[102] as indicated in Fig 10-2.

Treatment Plan

Alveolar bone fracture

Reposition the displaced teeth and alveolar bone at the same time. Use teeth for splinting. Remove the splint 2 to 3 months later.

Fracture of maxillary or mandibular diaphysis

Treatment of patients with complex injuries such as fractures of the maxilla and mandible should be referred to specialists in oral and maxillofacial surgery.

Treatment Procedures

1. *Examination and diagnosis*: Where there is trauma to multiple teeth and post-trauma malposition of teeth, even if there is no obvious luxation, bone fracture should be suspected (Figs 10-4a to f) and radiographs made. Examine the entire jaw with pantomography.
2. *Repositioning, suturing, and splinting*: After the administration of anesthetic, reposition the teeth and alveolar bone. Attend to any other problems related to the trauma, and suture the soft tissue and splint the teeth (Fig 10-4g).
3. *Endodontic treatment*: Traumatized teeth associated with alveolar bone fracture usually have apical vascular disruption of the pulps. Perform endodontic treatment for pulp necrosis (Fig 10-4h) so that it does not hinder fracture healing.
4. *Removal of splint and follow-up*: Two to 3 months later, remove splint and confirm healing clinically and radiographically. Periodically monitor the progress of healing (Figs 10-4i to l).

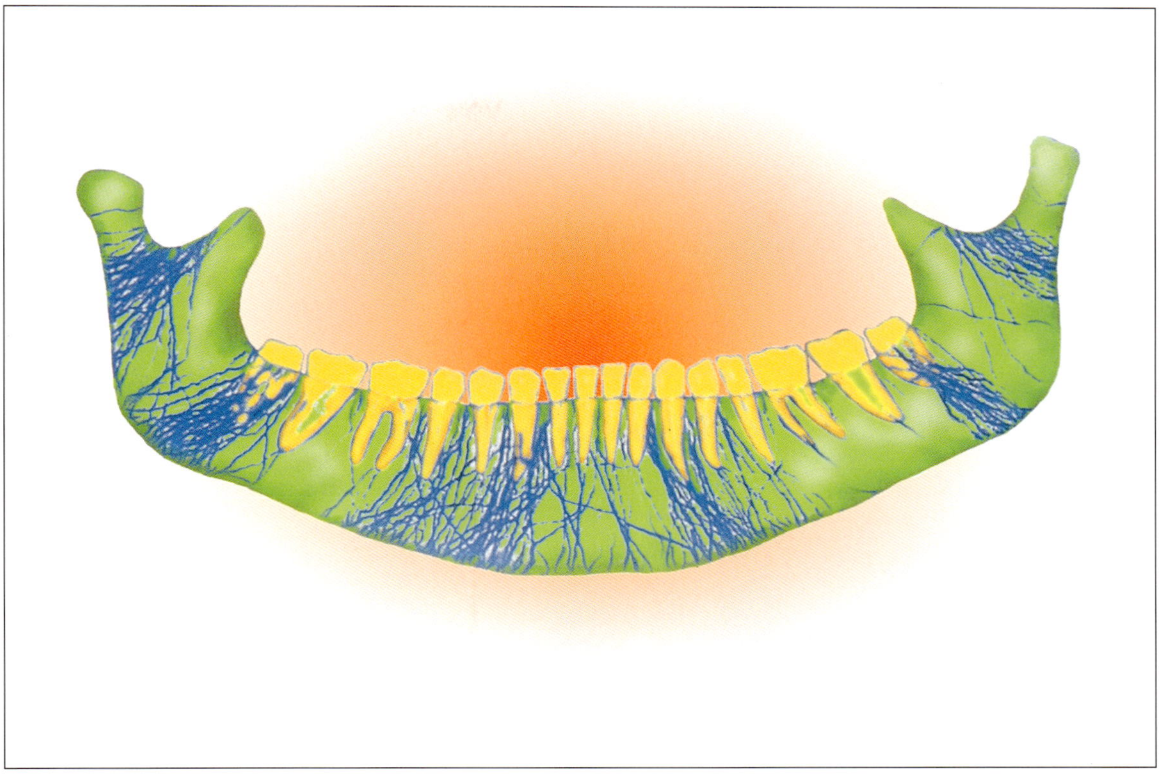

Fig 10-2 Mandibular bone fracture and areas of predilection.[102] Reprinted from Andreasen and Andreasen.[7]

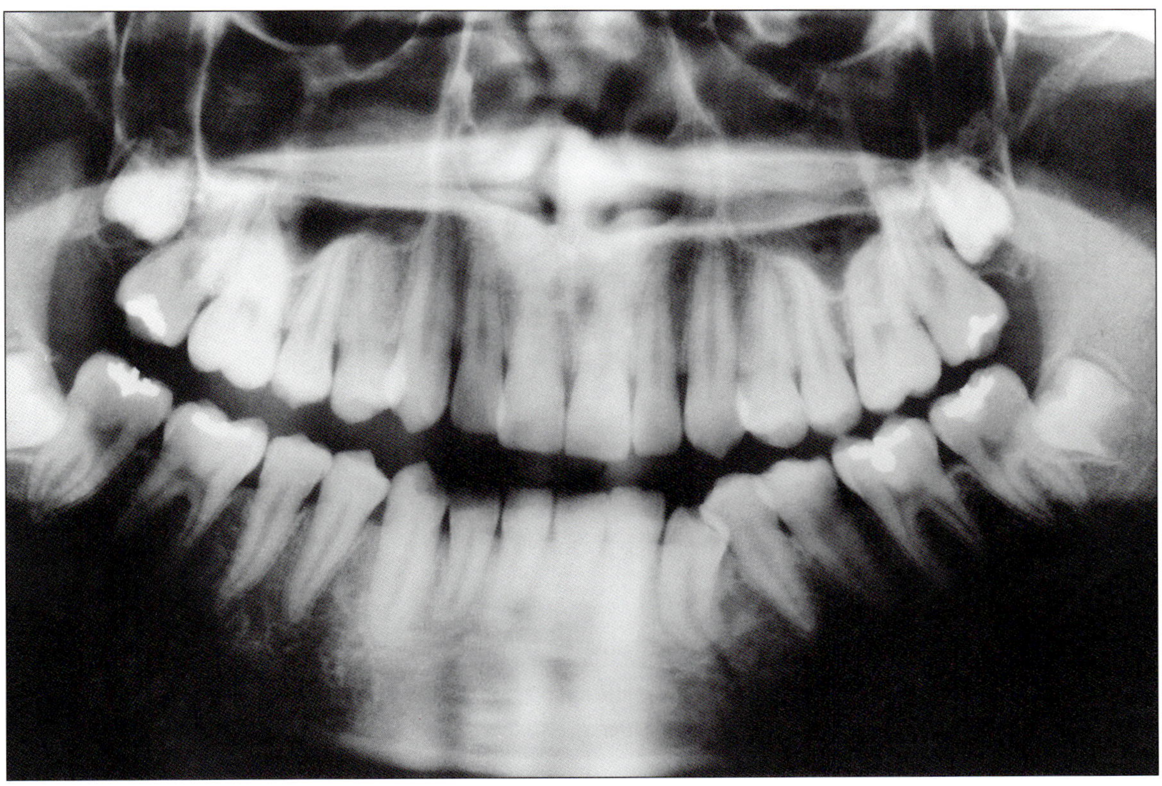

Fig 10-3 Mandibular bone fracture. A 15-year-old girl has malocclusion and left facial swelling. Note fracture of the diaphysis in the area of tooth 22.

Fig 10-4 Treatment procedures for alveolar bone fracture

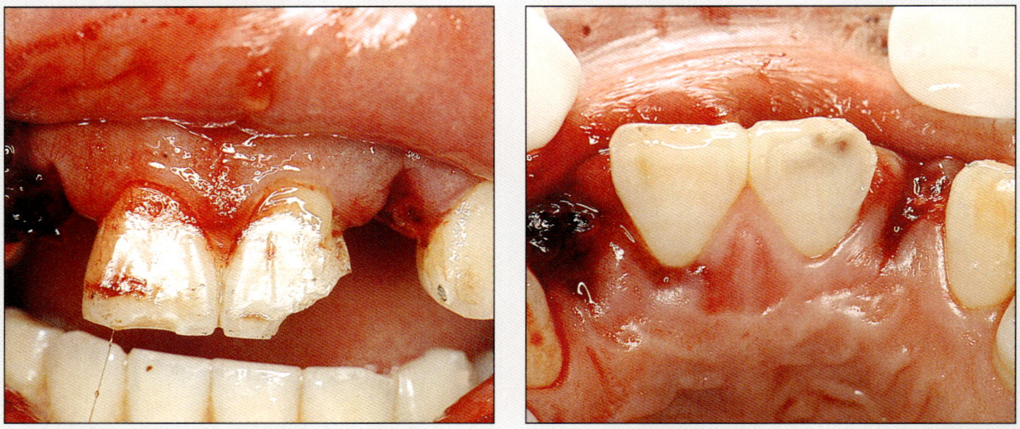

Figs10-4a and b Initial examination. Seventeen-year-old boy 12 hours after a fall from a motorcycle.

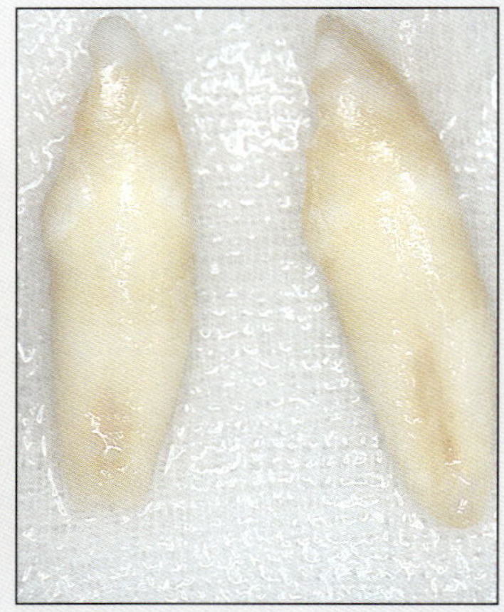

Fig 10-4c The avulsed teeth (7 and 10) remained at the site of the accident for 12 hours.

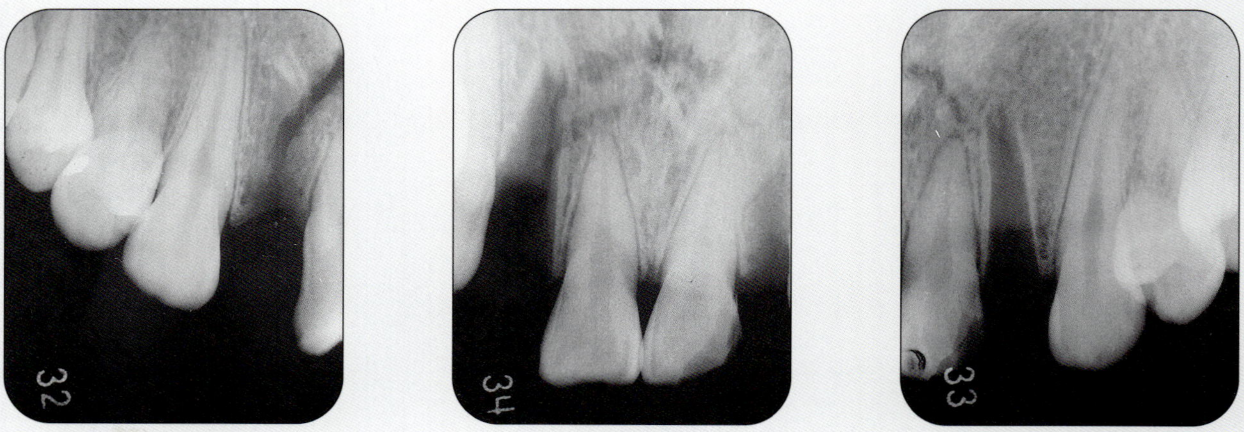

Figs 10-4d to f Radiographs at initial examination. Note the fracture line.

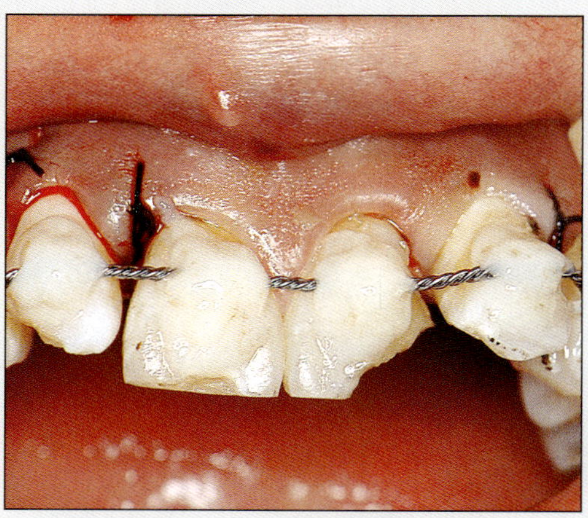

Fig10-4g Teeth 7 and 10 were replanted, the alveolar segment containing teeth 8 and 9 was repositioned, and a splint was placed and the soft tissue sutured.

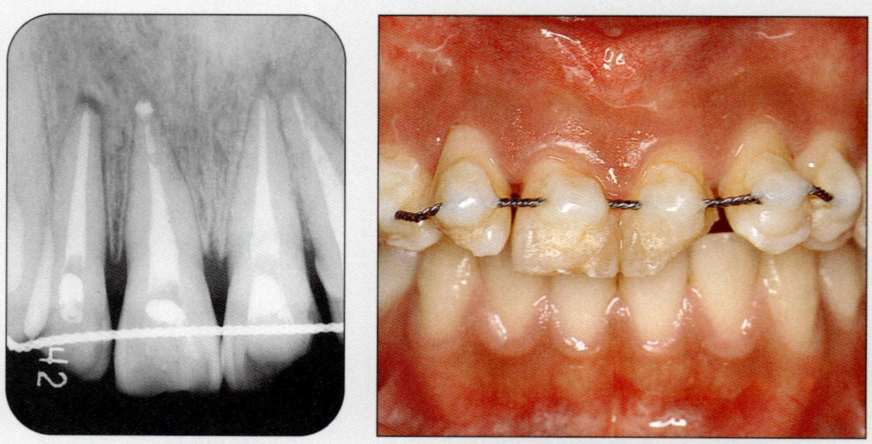

Figs 10-4h and i After 6 weeks. Teeth 8 and 9 underwent endodontic treatment because of signs of pulp necrosis. A calcium hydroxide preparation was used for root canal filling. Endodontic treatment was performed on teeth 7 and 10 immediately after replantation.

Fig 10-4 (Continued)

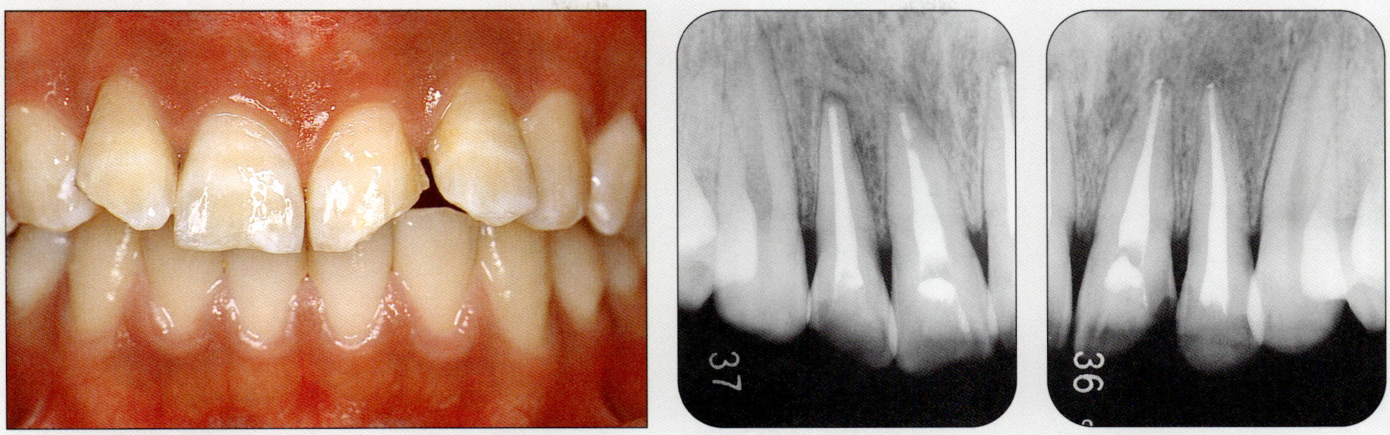

Figs 10-4j to l Six months later, the fracture has healed. Replanted teeth 7 and 10 healed by ankylosis.

Trauma to the Gingiva and Alveolar Mucosa: Description

Abrasion

An abrasion is a superficial wound in which the epithelial tissue is rubbed or scratched (Fig 10-5).

Contusion

A contusion is hemorrhage of subcutaneous tissue without laceration of epithelial tissue. It is usually caused by a blunt object hitting the tissue (Fig 10-6).

Laceration

A laceration is the tearing of tissue usually caused by a sharp object (Figs 10-7 to 10-10).

Examination and Diagnosis: Key Points

Perform inspection and palpation to confirm the size and depth of the injury and the degree of bleeding. Especially in lacerated areas, check for embedded fragments of teeth and foreign bodies. Radiographic examination aids in disclosing foreign body impaction.

Treatment Plan

For abrasions and contusions, only cleansing and observation are necessary. For lacerations, depending on their size and depth, suture the wounds after the administration of local anesthetic (Fig 10-11).

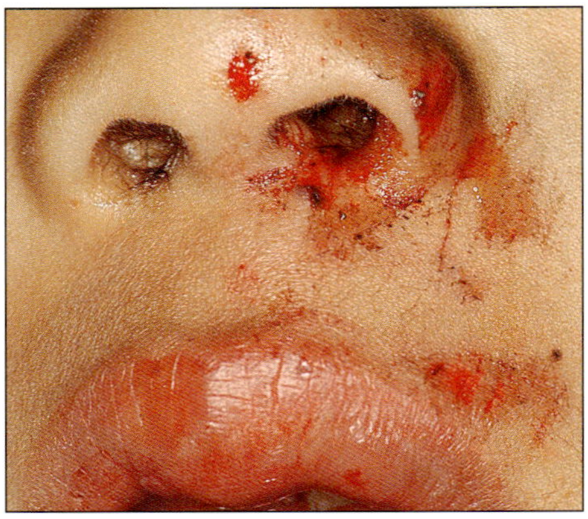

Fig 10-5 Abrasion.

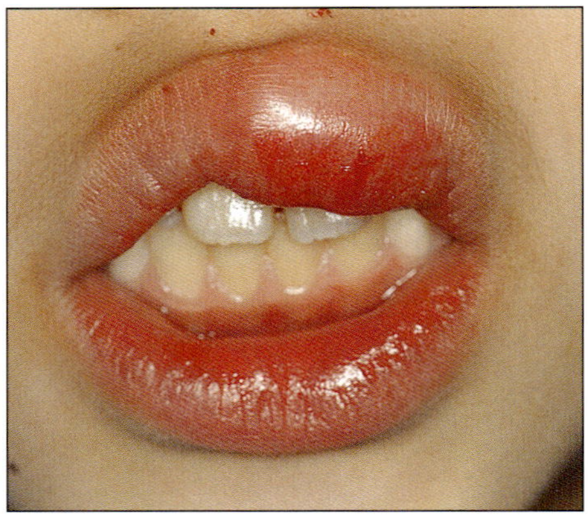

Fig 10-6 Contusion.

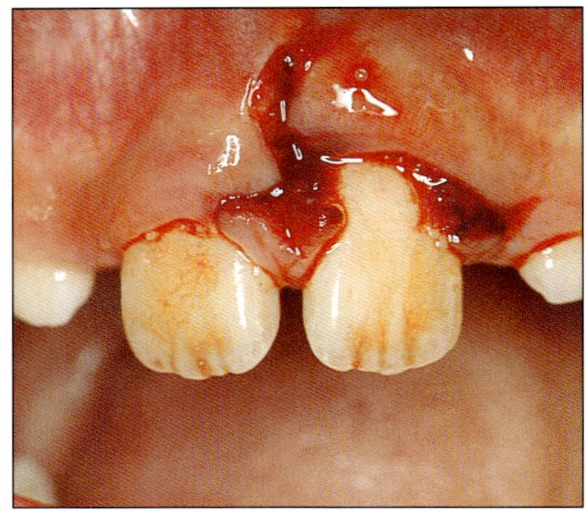

Fig 10-7 Laceration.

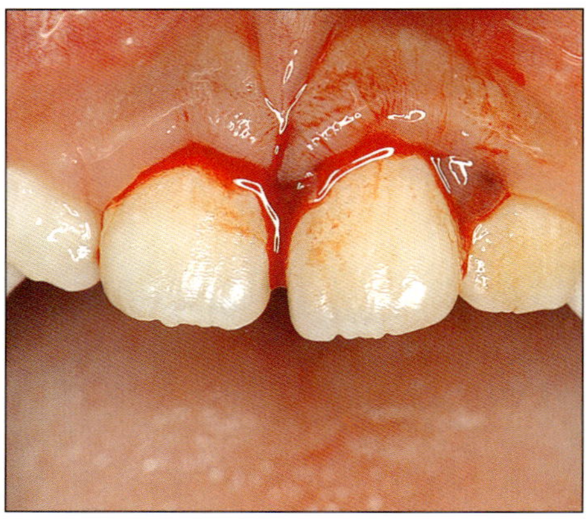

Fig 10-8 Laceration of the gingival sulcus caused by pulling of the frenum of the upper lip.

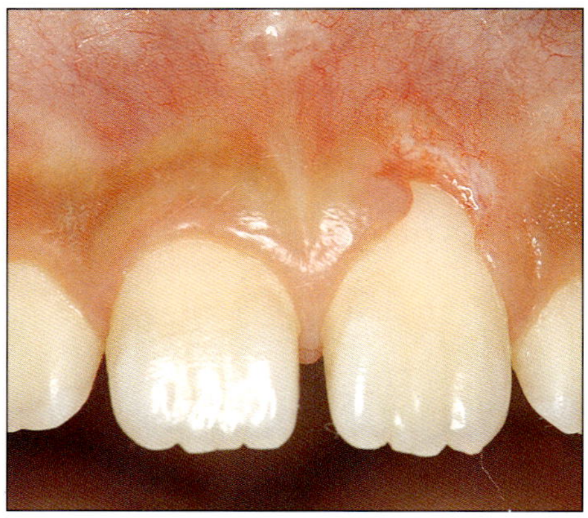

Fig 10-9 Dehiscence defect of the gingiva expected to heal naturally.

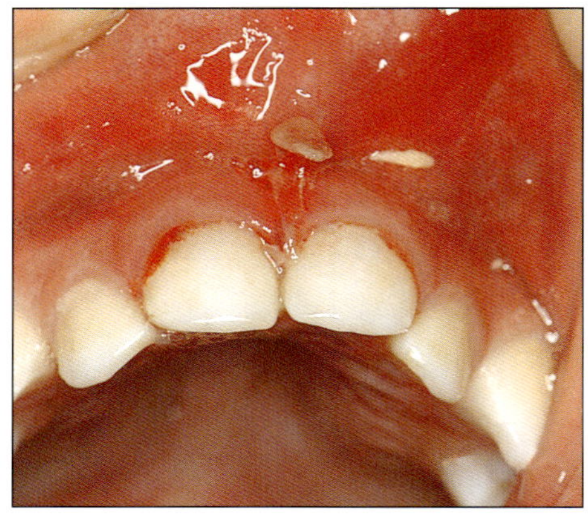

Fig 10-10 Laceration of the frenum is often observed in children. Treatment is unnecessary.

Fig 10-11 Treatment plan for laceration

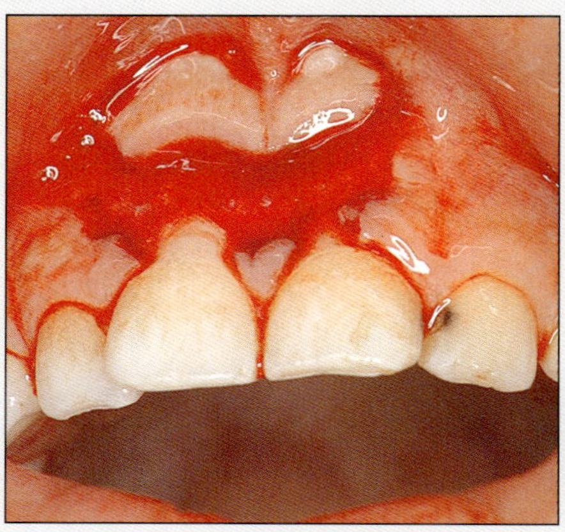

Fig 10-11a Preoperative view. The gingiva is stripped from the periosteum.

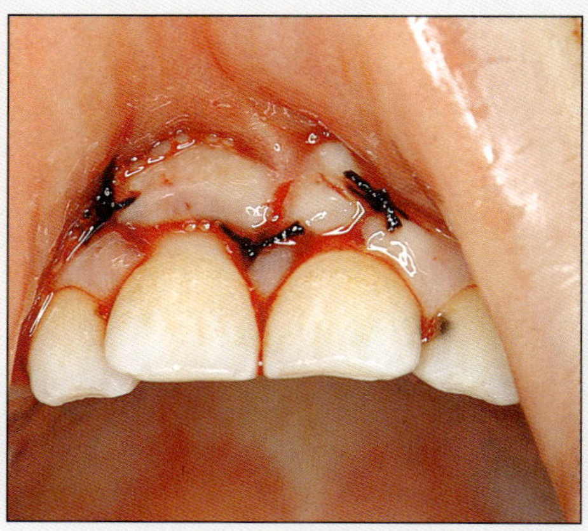

Fig 10-11b A suture is made after the administration of anesthetic.

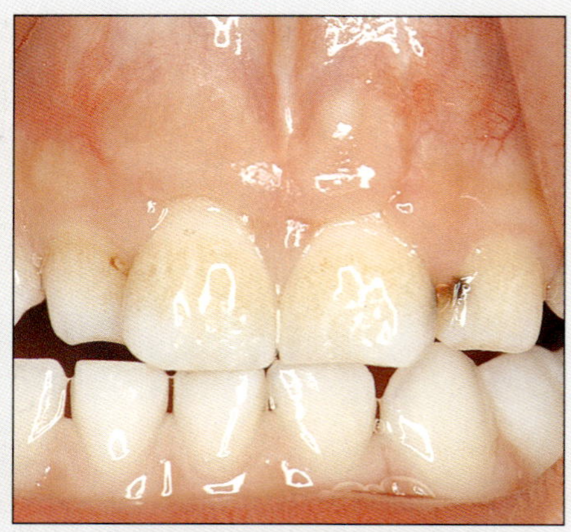

Fig 10-11c After healing.

11

Trauma to the Primary Dentition

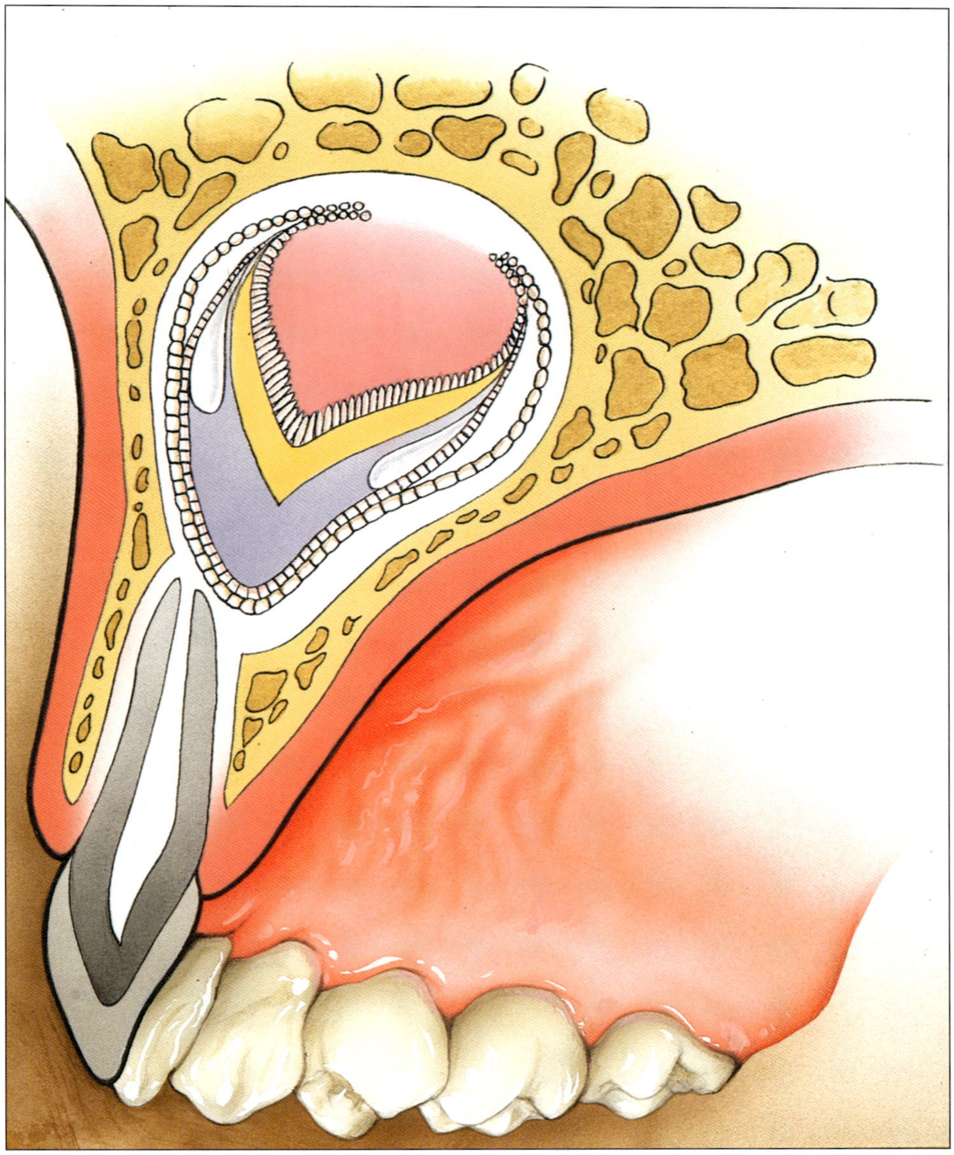

When trauma involves the primary dentition, concern must be directed to both the teeth involved and the subjacent developing permanent dentition. Every effort must be made to protect the developing tooth buds, and treatment plans must be thus prepared.

Description

One of the problems of trauma to the primary dentition is the possibility of damaging the permanent successor tooth buds[103,104] (Fig 11-1). The patient's age and the degree and direction of the malposition of the primary teeth are some of the factors. Possible sequelae to permanent teeth following trauma involving primary teeth include:

1. Discoloration and hypoplasia of the enamel (Fig 11-2)
2. Bending and malformation of the anatomic crown and root (Fig 11-3)
3. Hypoplasia of the root
4. Retarded eruption

These problems may occur regardless of the treatment of the traumatized primary teeth. It is important to inform patients' parents about these possibilities and to try to resolve the problems at the time the primary teeth are being replaced with permanent teeth. Periodic examinations are essential. Hypoplasia of the enamel can be restored after eruption (Fig 11-2), and bending and malformation of the crown and root may be treated with orthodontic and restorative procedures.

Examination and Diagnosis: Key Points

Primary tooth injuries include: crown fracture (with or without pulp exposure), crown-root fracture, root fracture, subluxation, lateral luxation, intrusive luxation, and avulsion. Examining and diagnosing children's teeth can be difficult. Because accurate radiographs may be difficult to obtain, an assistant's help may be required. If the film holder cannot be used, use a finger to hold the film toward the palatal (lingual) aspect, and reduce the radiation time to one-half to two-thirds of the adult dose. For a cooperative child, the electric pulp test may be useful for checking the vitality of the pulp.

Treatment Plan

The treatment plan for primary teeth is usually different from that for permanent teeth. The reasons are: the healing mechanism of pulp and periodontal tissues in primary teeth is different than that of permanent teeth, healing observed in permanent teeth may not be expected in primary teeth, sometimes extraction has priority to limit damage to permanent successors, and treatment may be impossible due to uncooperative behavior. A lack of understanding of the healing mechanism unique to primary teeth may result in unnecessary treatment or extraction.

Discolored primary teeth

Occasionally parents complain about discoloration of their children's primary teeth or discoloration may go unnoticed. Discoloration of primary teeth may be caused by slight damage, such as concussion and subluxation. The discoloration usually occurs within 2 months after trauma.

In discolored primary teeth, it is best to first observe without treatment. In many cases, the discoloration will be reduced with time as pulp obliteration occurs (Fig 11-4). Obliteration usually occurs within 6 months after discoloration is first observed. Pulp obliteration may also be observed without any reduction in discoloration (Fig 11-5). Because pulp obliteration is pulp healing, treatment is unnecessary.

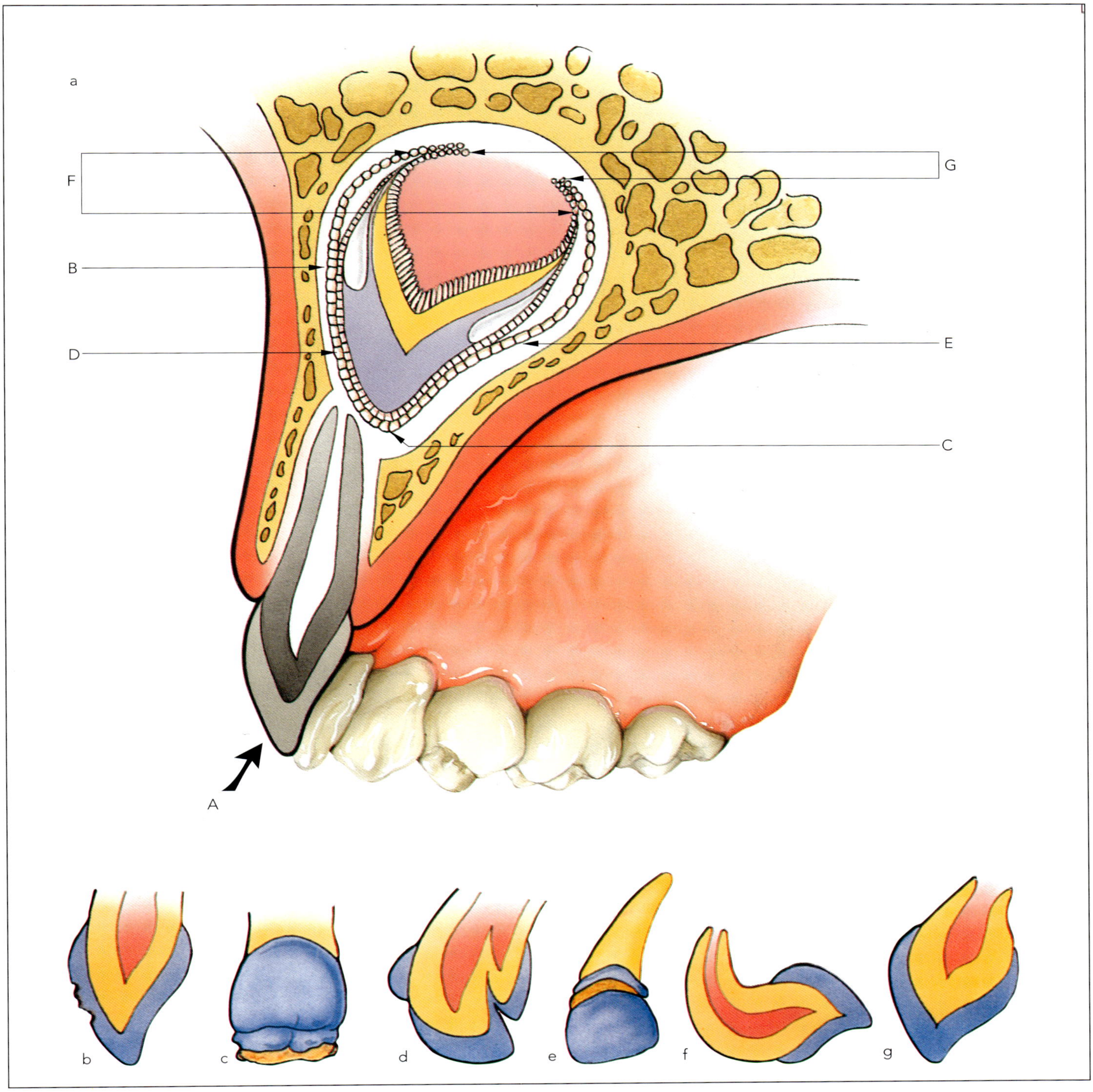

Fig 11-1 Speculative effects of trauma to the primary teeth on permanent tooth buds.[7] (a) The position where the traumatic force (A) is delivered to permanent tooth germ. (b) Buccal intrusion of the primary tooth damages the enamel and enamel organ during formation (B), resulting in hypoplasia and pigmentation. (c) Malformation of the crown and hypoplasia of the enamel are due to vertical force on C early in development. (d and e) Bending and deformity of the crown is caused by the tooth germ being bent between E and B due to the root of the primary tooth being pushed against the tooth germ palatally at D. (f) Bending of the root is caused by the tooth germ being bent at F. (g) Lack of root development is caused by damage to Hertwig's epithelial root sheath when the entire tooth germ is pushed apically.

Fig 11-2 Malformation of the anatomic crown

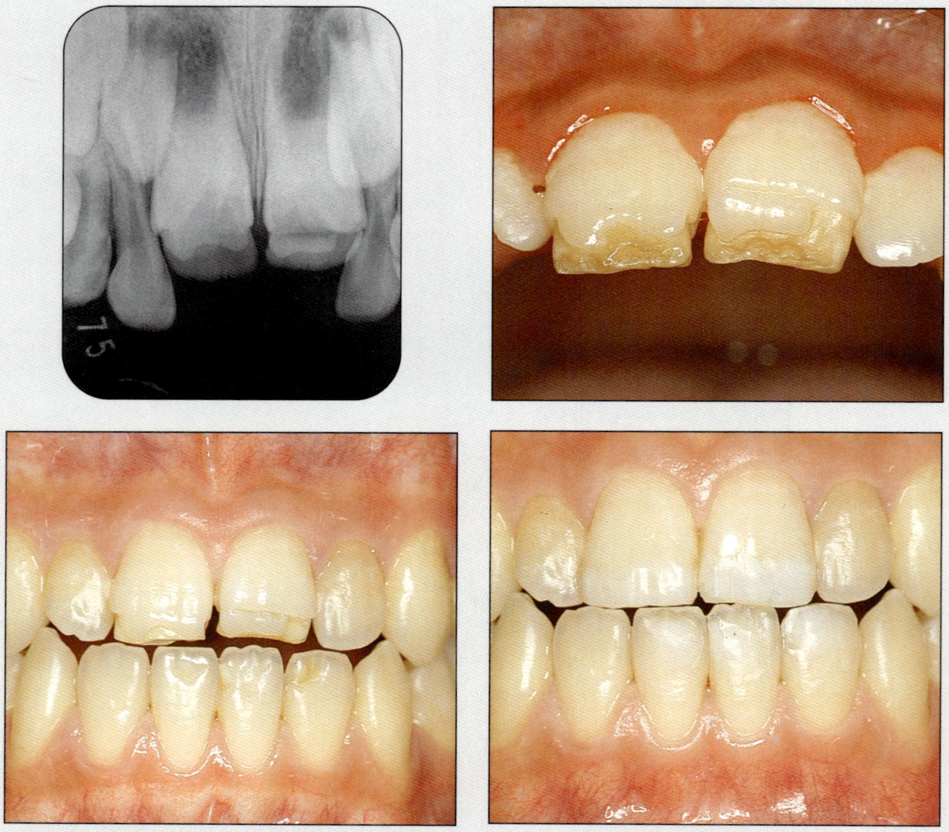

Fig 11-2a Before eruption of teeth 8 and 9.

Fig 11-2b After eruption of teeth 8 and 9. Note malformation of the crowns.

Fig 11-2c Five years after eruption. The teeth are sufficiently mature to undergo treatment.

Fig 11-2d After restorative treatment using composite resin.

Fig 11-3 Curvature of root

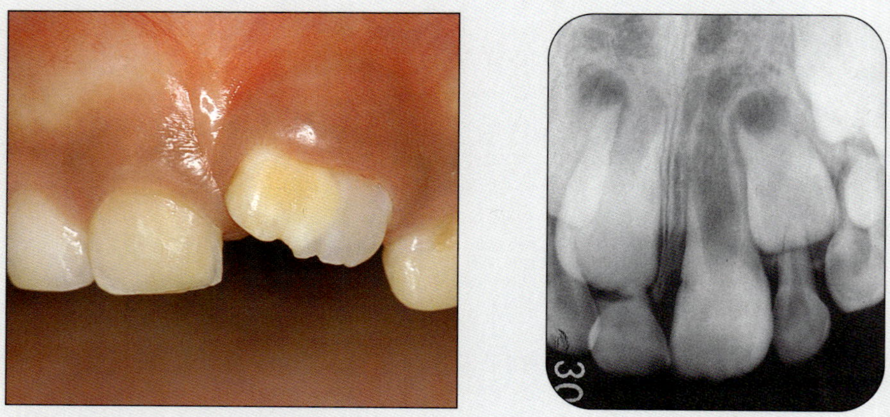

Fig 11-3a Note the pigmentation (hypoplasia) and curvature of the crown of tooth 9 after eruption.

Fig 11-3b Note the radiolucency on the mesial part of the curvature due to hypoplasia.

The primary teeth will soon be replaced by permanent teeth. However, if discoloration continues without pulp obliteration, there is a possibility of pulp necrosis. If there is a gingival abscess or subjective symptoms, endodontic treatment or extraction is indicated (Fig 11-6).

Fig 11-4 Treatment for discolored primary tooth—case 1

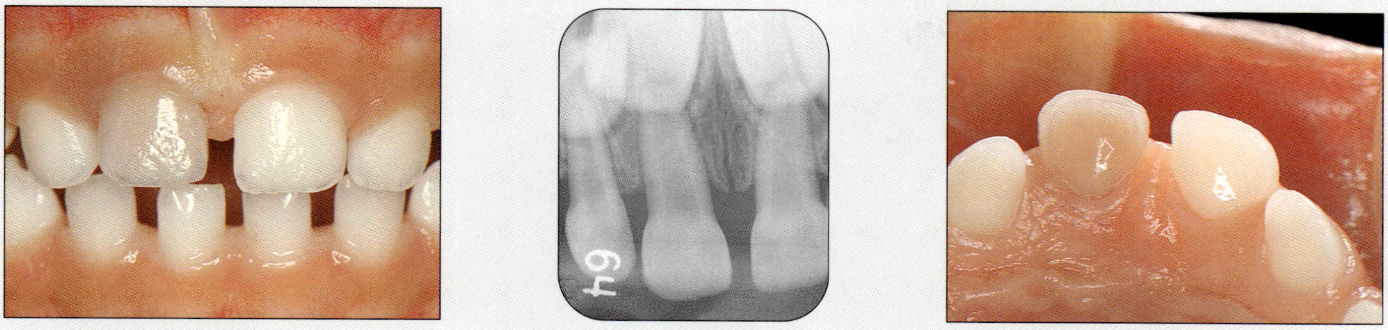

Figs 11-4a to c Initial examination, 4-year-old girl. Chief complaint: discoloration of tooth E. Subluxation 1 to 2 months earlier is suspected.

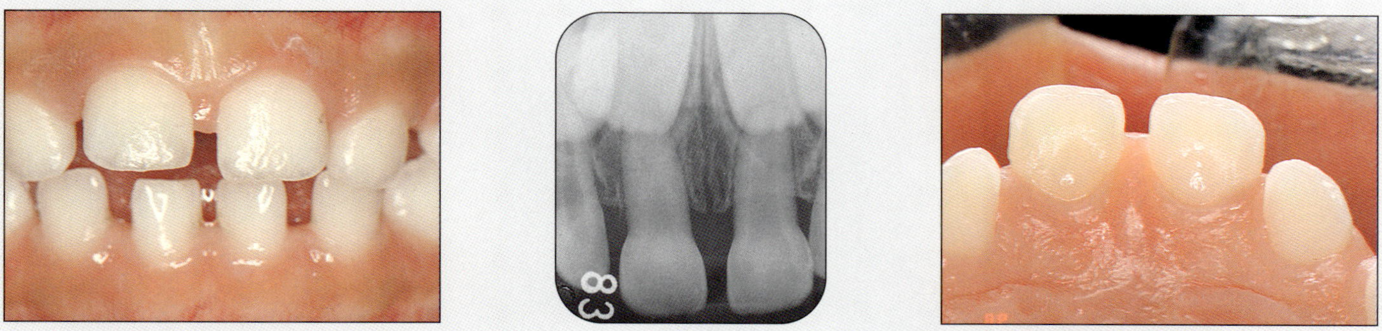

Figs 11-4d to f Six months later. No discoloration of tooth E. Also note pulp obliteration. Treatment is unnecessary.

Fig 11-5 Treatment for discolored primary tooth—case 2

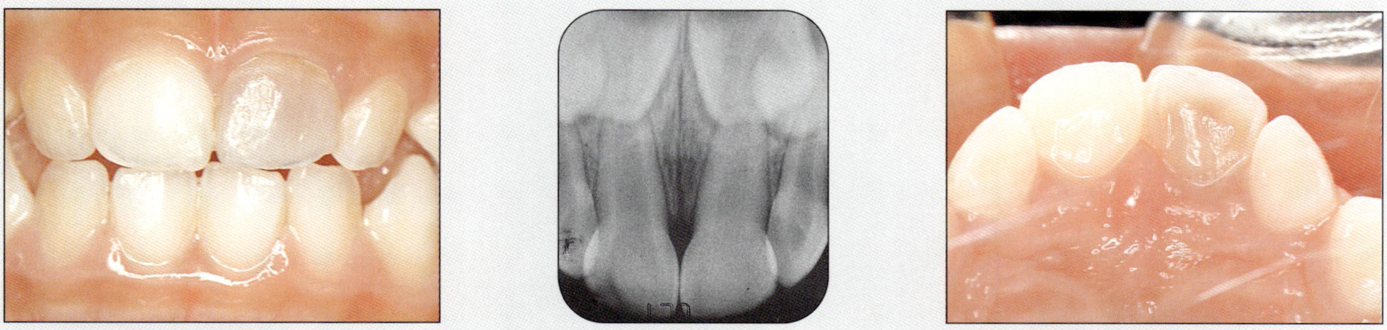

Figs 11-5a to c Initial examination, 3-year-old girl. Chief complaint: discoloration of tooth F. Pulp obliteration is in progress.

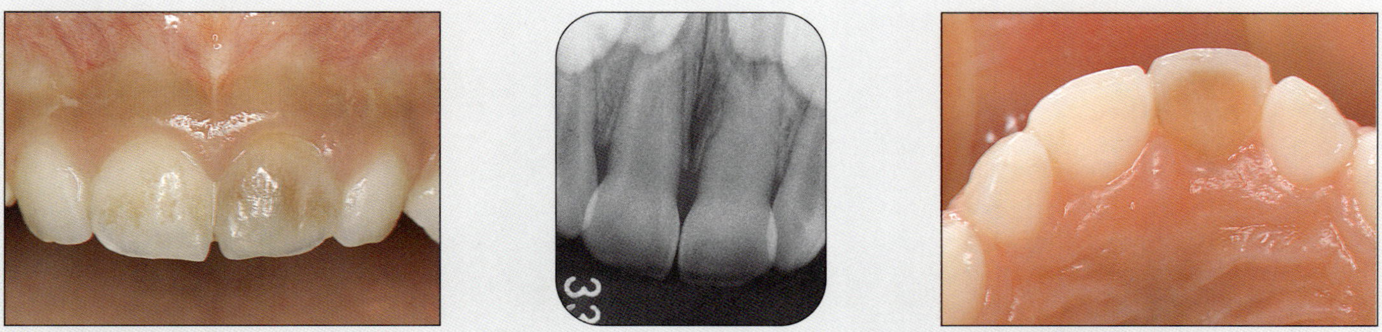

Figs 11-5d to f Two years and 8 months later. Discoloration of tooth F has continued, but the pulp cavity is obliterated. Treatment is unnecessary.

Fig 11-6 Treatment for discolored primary teeth—case 3

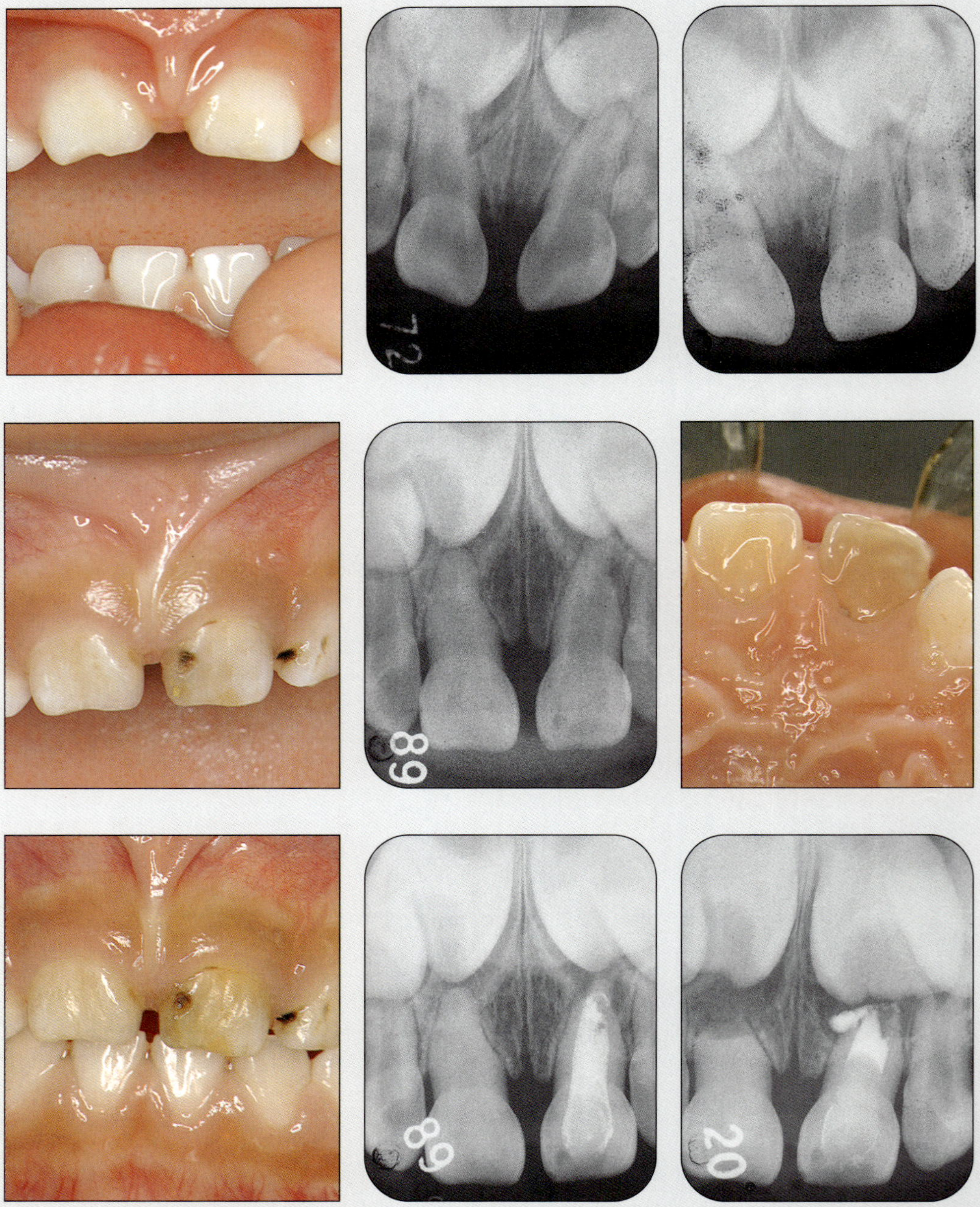

Figs 11-6a and b Initial examination, 2-year, 2-month-old girl. Chief complaint: concussion of anterior teeth. Neither discoloration nor obliteration is observed.

Fig 11-6c Three months later. There is no change in the pulp cavities.

Figs 11-6d to f Two years and 3 months later. Note discoloration of the crown of tooth F and a small facial abscess. Obliteration of the pulp cavity is not observed in this tooth but can be seen in the adjacent tooth E, which is not discolored.

Figs 11-6g and h Two years and 10 months later. Seven months after endodontic treatment of tooth F.

Fig 11-6i Four years later, immediately after retreatment of tooth F. A delay is expected in the root resorption of tooth F.

Crown fracture without pulp exposure

Selectively grind to correct the sharp edges without restorative treatment. Should there be pain to cold, use glass-ionomer cement for pulp protection on the fractured surface. If the young patient is cooperative and the parents desire restorative treatment, use composite resin.

Crown fracture and crown-root fracture with pulp exposure

In a case of pulp exposure of primary teeth due to a crown fracture, perform pulp extirpation and root canal treatment (Fig 11-7).

Fig 11-7 Treatment plan for crown-root fracture of primary tooth

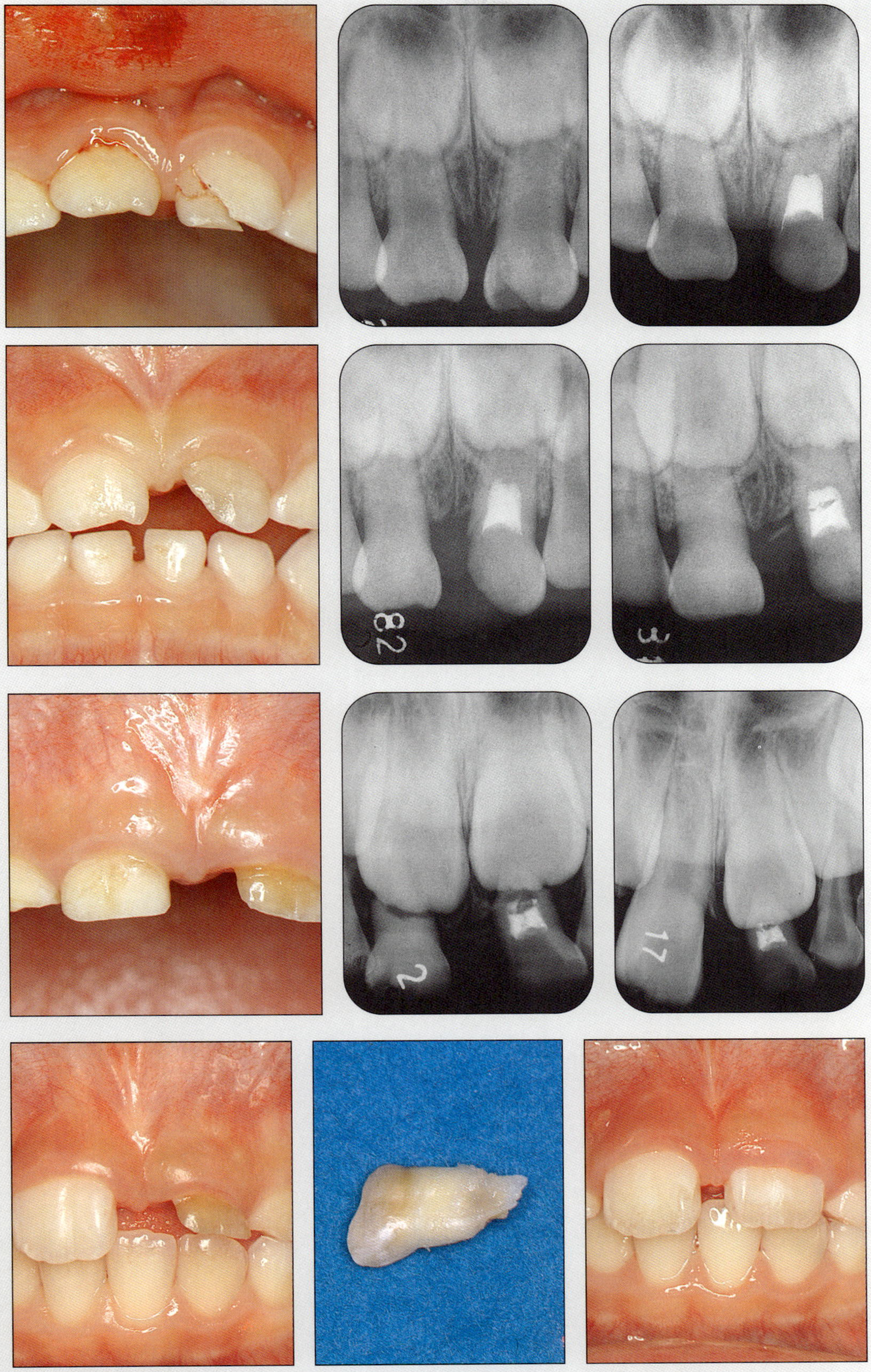

Figs 11-7a and b Initial examination, 2-year, 7-month-old boy. Crown-root fracture with pulp exposure can be seen in tooth F.

Fig 11-7c After root canal treatment. Calcium hydroxide was used for root canal filling.

Figs 11-7d and e Four months later.

Fig 11-7f Two years later.

Figs 11-7g and h Four years and 4 months later.

Fig 11-7i Five years and 7 months later. Note the incomplete root resorption of tooth F.

Fig 11-7j After 5 years and 7 months. Tooth F was extracted that day.

Fig 11-7k Extracted tooth F.

Fig 11-7l Three months after extraction of tooth F. Tooth 9 is erupting and soon will be positioned similar to tooth 8.

Fig 11-8 Treatment of primary tooth with root fracture

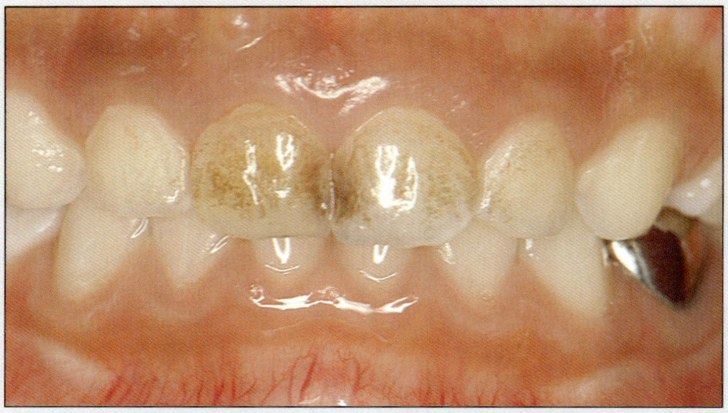

Figs 11-8a and b Initial examination, 5-year, 4-month-old girl. Chief complaint: gingival abscess labial to tooth E caused by root fracture.

Fig 11-8c After endodontic treatment of the coronal segment with calcium hydroxide.

Fig 11-8d One year later. The apical fragment of tooth E has been resorbed.

Fig 11-8e Radiograph 2 years later.

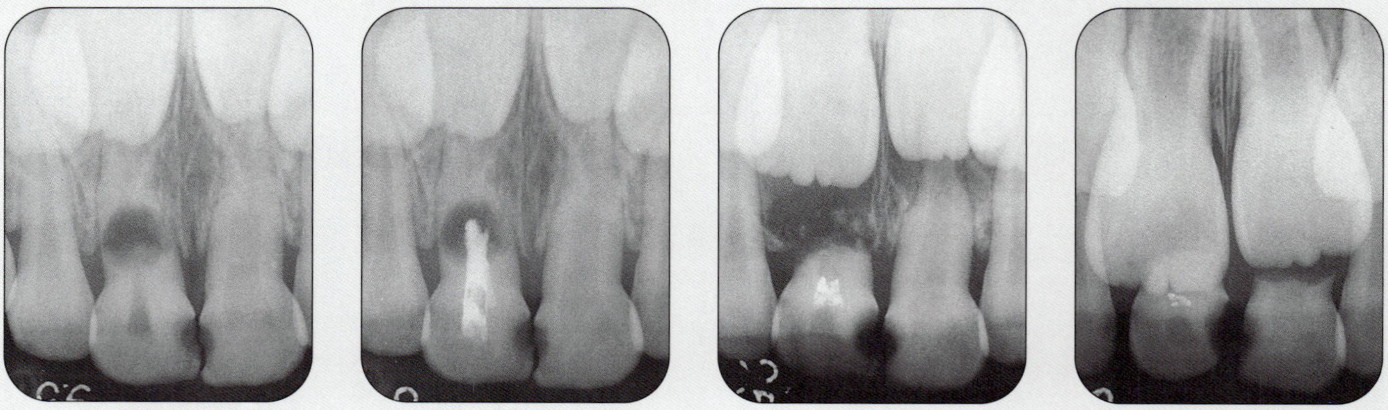

Root fracture

In a root fracture of primary teeth, treatment is unnecessary as long as infection does not occur. If rapid root resorption is observed at the fracture site, remove only the coronal portion or perform root canal treatment of the coronal portion because necrosis of the coronal pulp is suspected. It is unnecessary to remove the fractured apical segment, because it will be resorbed naturally (Fig 11-8).

Concussion and subluxation

If neither malpositioning of the teeth nor bleeding is observed after trauma to primary teeth, usually concussion or subluxation is the diagnosis, and discoloration of the crowns or pulp obliteration may be seen after the injury (see Figs 11-4 and 11-5). Inform parents of these possibilities even if no abnormality is apparent and emphasize the importance of observation and periodic examinations.

Extrusive, lateral, and intrusive luxation

Reposition the dislocated injured primary teeth, then allow natural healing to take place (Fig 11-9). This is done to avoid further traumatic force against the permanent tooth buds. The author usually performs repositioning and suturing of the gingiva and splinting of the teeth as with permanent teeth (Fig 11-10). Special attention to the direction of force is required to avoid additional mechanical trauma to the permanent tooth buds. There is usually pulp obliteration or rapid root resorption after treatment, whether or not treatment (repositioning and splinting) is performed (Figs 11-9 and 11-10). Treatment is usually unnecessary in cases of obliteration or resorption; however, explain to the parents what might occur subsequently.

Fig 11-9 Treatment of primary tooth displacement—case 1

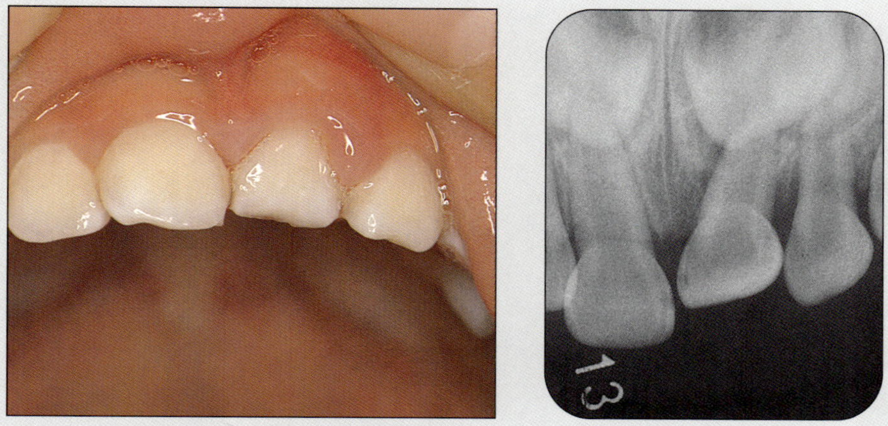

Figs 11-9a and b Initial examination of a 3-year-old boy with intrusive luxation of tooth F.

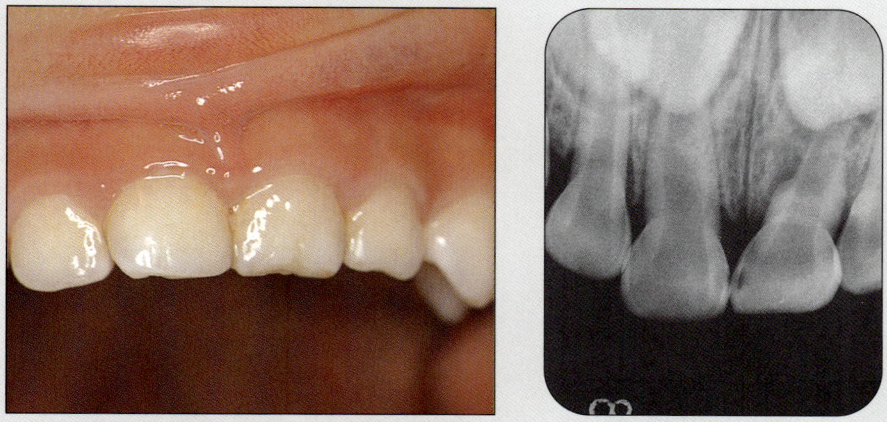

Figs 11-9c and d Three months later. No treatment is given while waiting for the natural eruption of the permanent tooth. Note the beginning of root resorption.

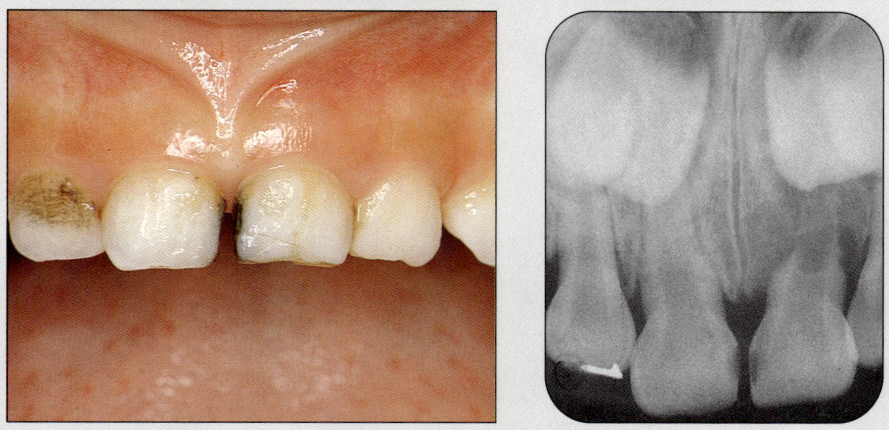

Figs 11-9e and f One year and 3 months later. Note obvious root resorption of tooth F. Continued observation is indicated.

Avulsion

Avulsed primary teeth in which the roots have begun normal resorption are not indicated for replantation. There is little value in replantation because of rapid root resorption or infection after trauma (or replantation). However, in young patients, the absence of teeth until the eruption of permanent teeth may cause esthetic and functional complications, and anxiety for themselves and their parents. Therefore, attempting replantation is sometimes worthwhile (Fig 11-11). Unlike permanent teeth, with replantation of primary teeth, healing of the pulp and periodontal membrane should not be expected. Furthermore, it is necessary to consider the risk of

Fig 11-10 Treatment of primary teeth displacement—case 2

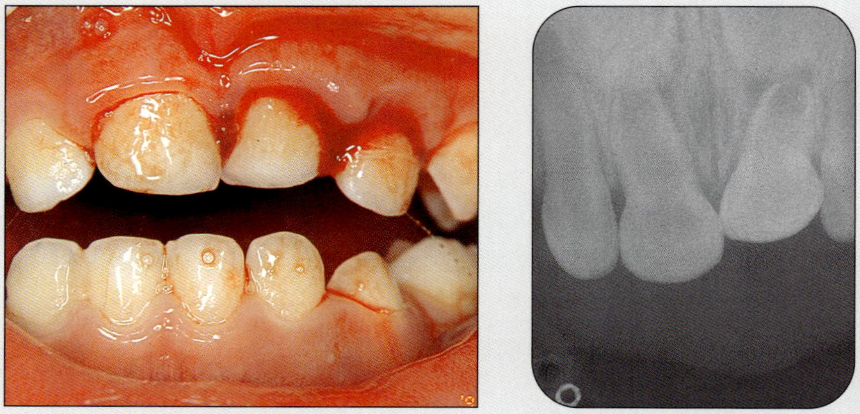

Figs 11-10a and b Initial examination, 1-year, 5-month-old boy. Diagnosis: tooth F, intrusive luxation; tooth G, subluxation or extrusive luxation.

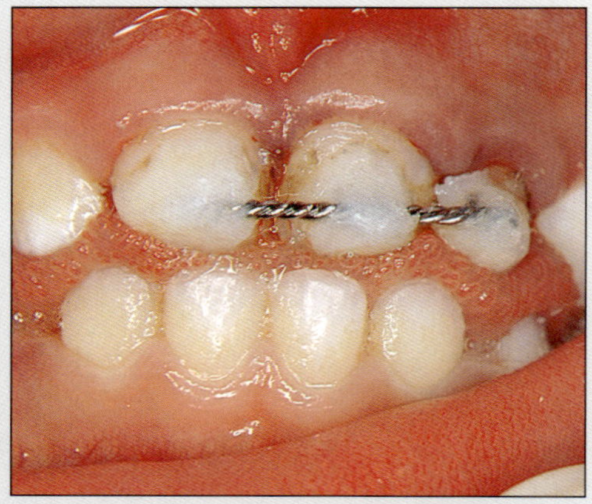

Fig 11-10c Repositioning and splinting was done after the administration of anesthetic.

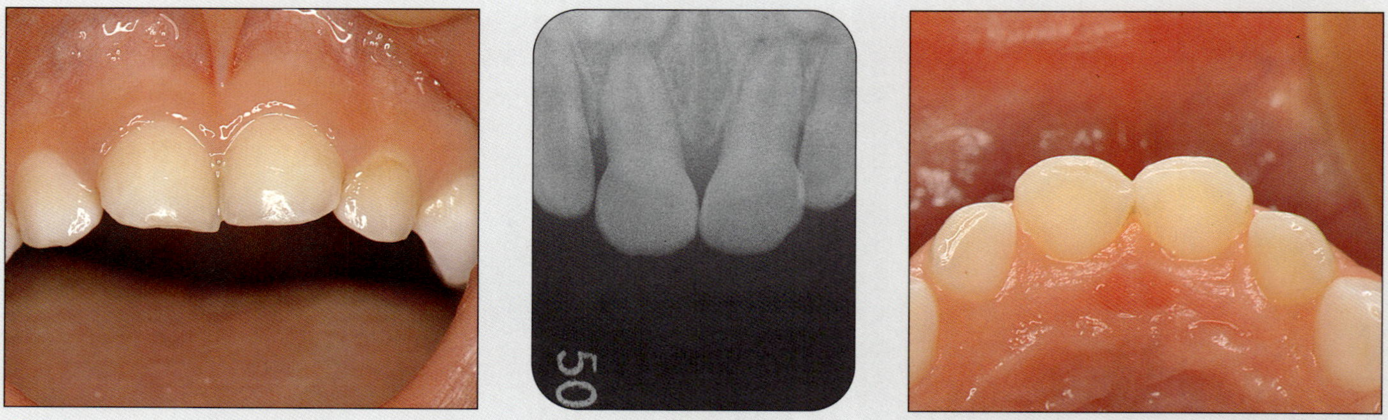

Figs 11-10d to f One year and 3 months later. Note the incomplete pulp obliteration.

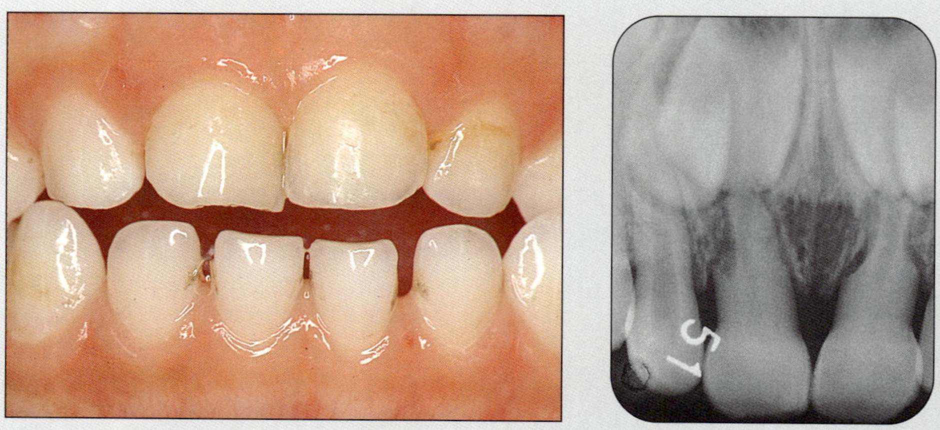

Figs 11-10g and h Two years and 3 months later. The beginning of vertical resorption is apparent, but it is not considered a problem.

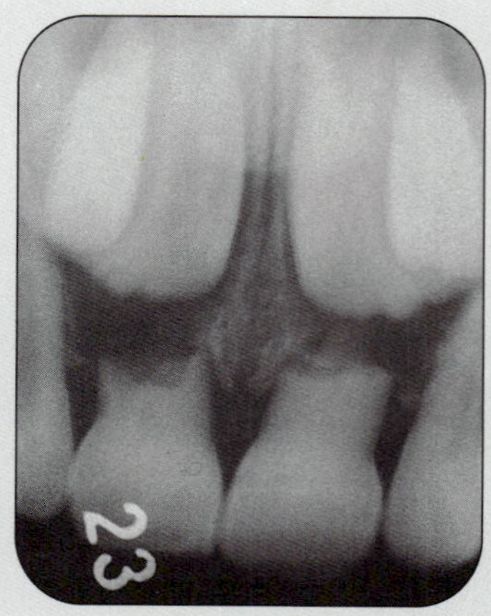

Fig 11-10i Three years and 7 months later. The pulp obliteration and accelerated root resorption are not considered problems.

Fig 11-11 Treatment of primary teeth avulsion

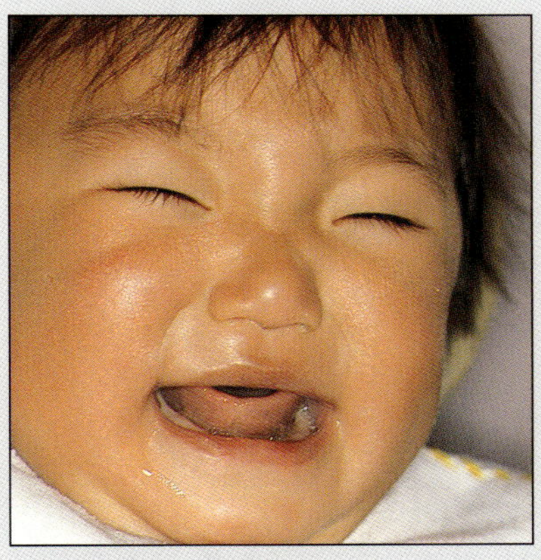

Fig 11-11a Initial examination of a 9-month-old girl with avulsion of teeth O and P.

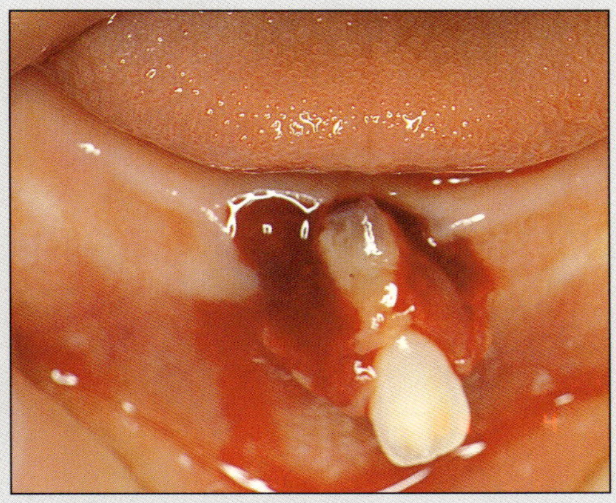

Fig 11-11b Tooth O in the oral cavity.

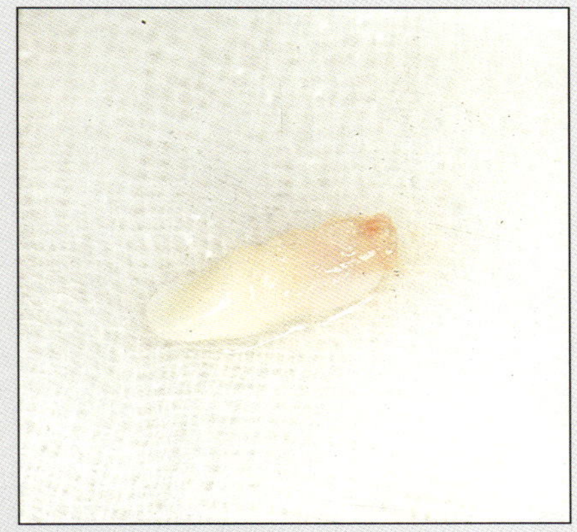

Fig 11-11c Tooth P. The initial visit is 15 minutes after injury.

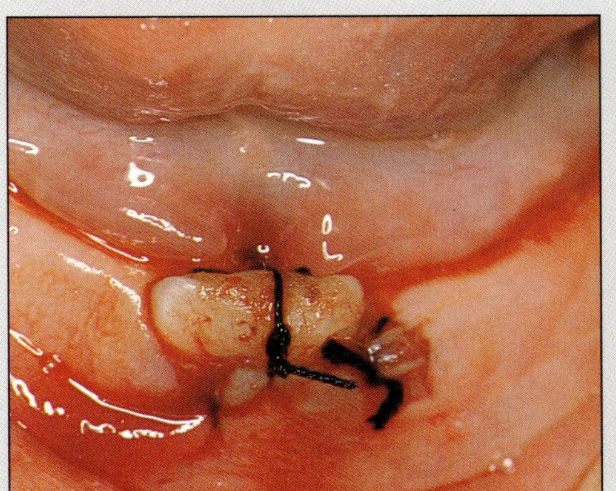

Fig 11-11d Immediately after replantation. A composite resin was used to splint teeth O and P, and the lacerated gingival tissues were sutured.

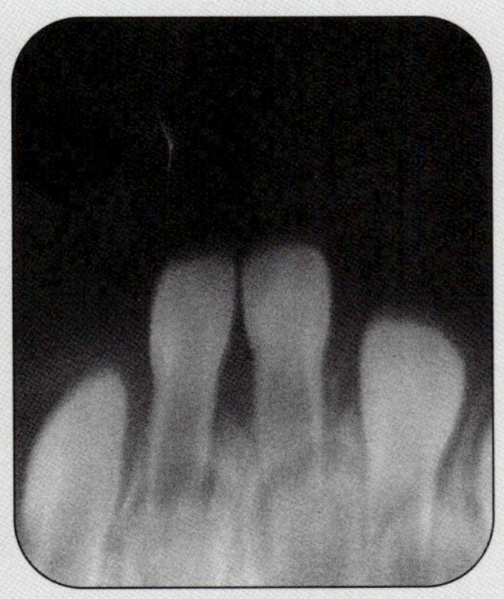

Fig 11-11e Two weeks later.

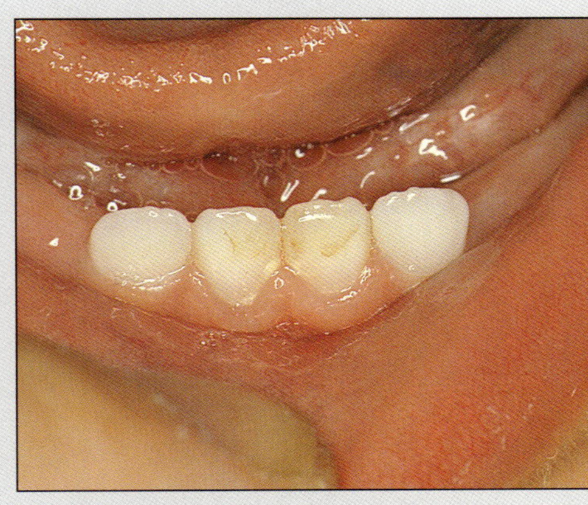

Fig 11-11f Four months later.

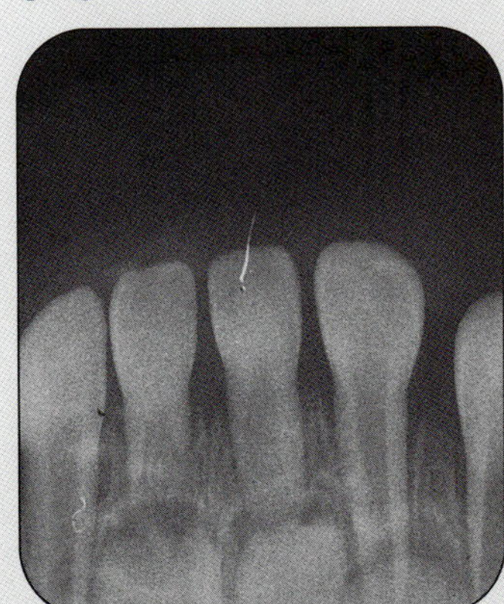

Fig 11-11g Eight months later.

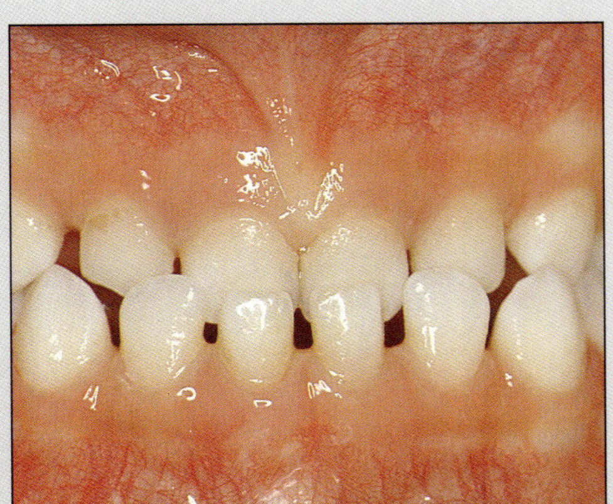

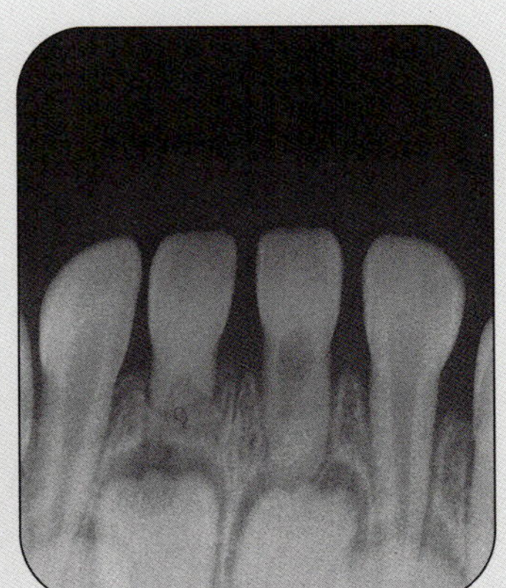

Figs 11-11h and i Two years and 3 months later.

damage to the permanent successor germ due to replantation. This is not the most desirable treatment plan; however, replantation may be considered if there is little risk of infection and damage to the permanent tooth bud.

Fig 11-11 (Continued)

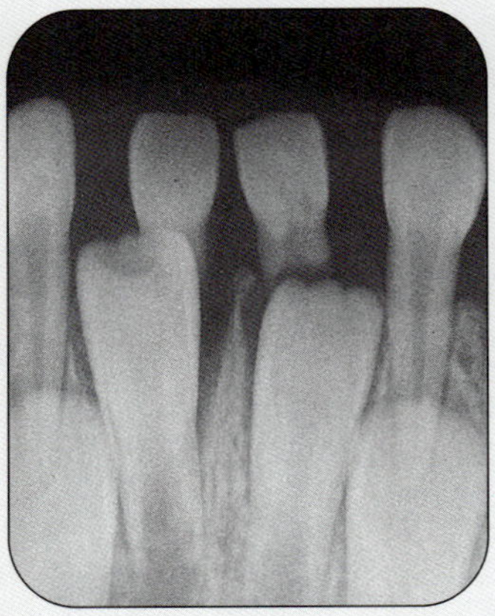

Fig 11-11j Three years and 10 months later.

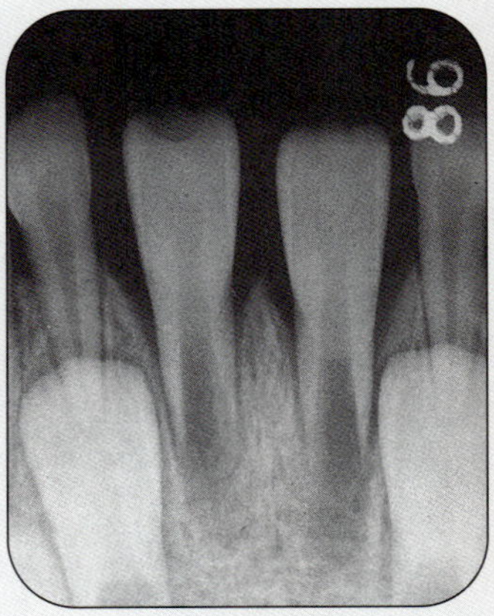

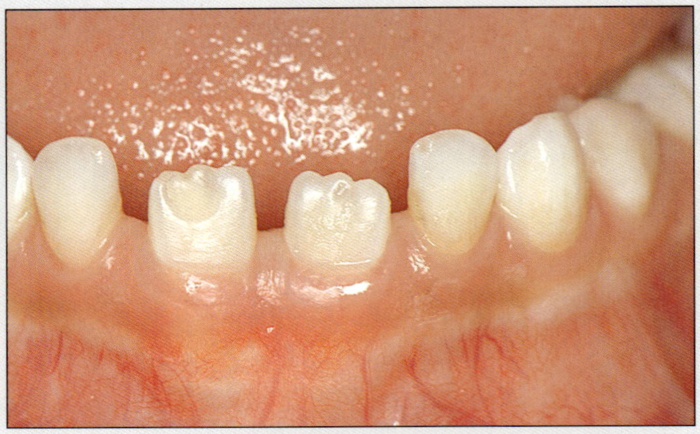

Figs 11-10k and l Four years and 1 month later. Note the small enamel defect on the facial aspect of tooth 25, which may have been caused by replantation of tooth P.

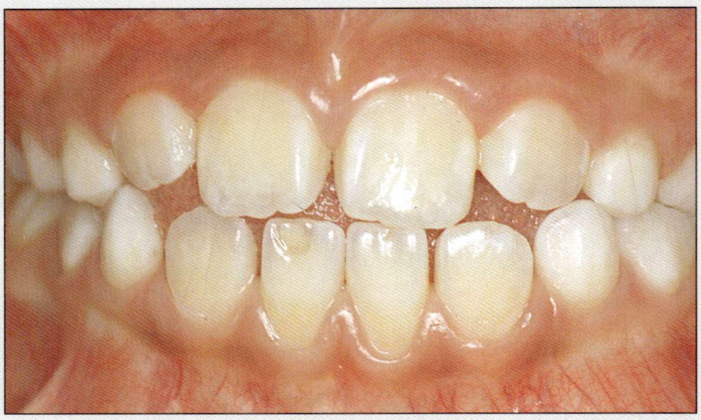

Fig 11-11m Five years and 7 months later.

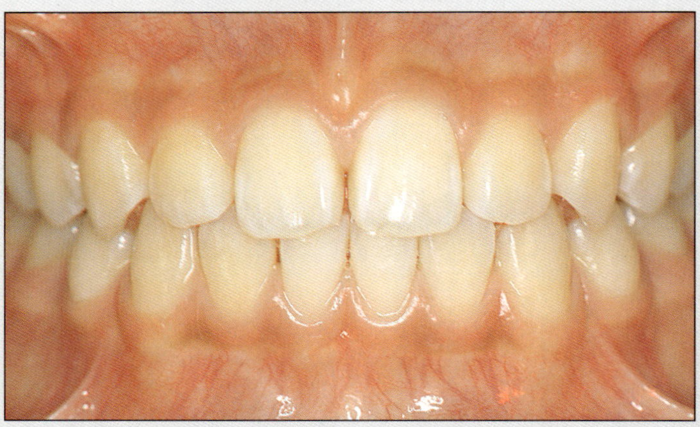

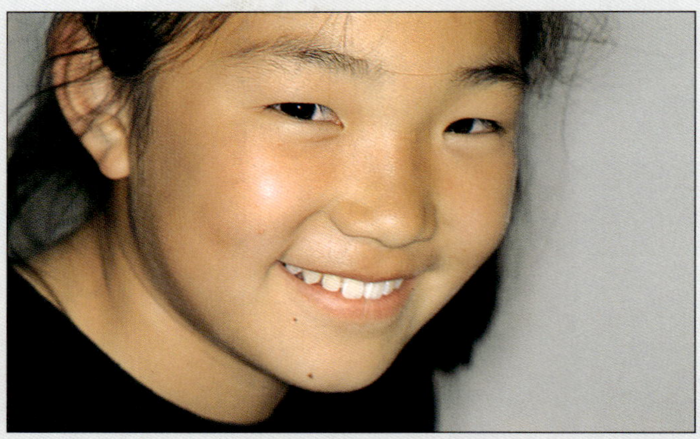

Figs 11-11n and o Nine years later. Successful replantation allowed the patient to have a normal dentition during her early development.

References

1. Ten Cate AR. Oral Histology, Development, Structure and Function, ed 3. St Louis: Mosby, 1989.
2. Bhaskar SN. Orban's Oral Histology and Embryology, ed 10. St Louis: Mosby, 1986.
3. Lindhe J. Textbook of Clinical Periodontology. Copenhagen: Munksgaard, 1984.
4. Ingber JS, Rose LF, Coslet JG. The "biologic width"—A concept in periodontics and restorative dentistry. Alpha Omegan 1977;70(3):62–65.
5. Andreasen JO. Traumatic Injuries of the Teeth, rev ed 2. Copenhagen: Munksgaard, 1981.
6. Andreasen JO, Andreasen FM. Essentials of Traumatic Injuries to the Teeth. Copenhagen: Munksgaard, 1990.
7. Andreasen JO, Andreasen FM. Textbook and Color Atlas of Traumatic Injuries to the Teeth, ed 3. Copenhagen: Munksgaard, 1994.
8. Simonsen RJ. Restoration of a fractured central incisor using original tooth fragment. J Am Dent Assoc 1982;105:648–650.
9. Shimono M, Maeda T, Suda H, et al. Dentin/Pulp Complex. Proceedings of the International Conference on Dentin/Pulp Complex 1995. Tokyo: Quintessence, 1996.
10. Cvek M. A clinical report on partial pulpotomy and capping with calcium hydroxide in permanent incisors with complicated crown fracture. J Endod 1978;4:232–237.
11. Cvek M, Lundberg M. Histological appearance of pulps after exposure by a crown fracture, partial pulpotomy, and clinical diagnosis of healing. J Endod 1983;9:8–11.
12. Nakabayashi N, Kojima K, Masuhara E. The promotion of adhesion by the infiltration of monomers into tooth substrates. J Biomed Mater Res 1982;16:265–273.
13. Nakabayashi N, Nakamura M, Yasuda N. Hybrid layer as a dentin-bonding mechanism. J Esthet Dent 1991;3:133–138.
14. Shimono M, Iijima K. Pathology of healing [in Japanese]. Tokyo: Ishiyaku Shuppan, 1993.
15. Inoue T, Enokiya Y, Shimono M, Miyakoshi S. A study of 4-META/MMA-TBB producing soft tissue hybrid layer. J Dent Res 1993;73(special issue):107.
16. Masaka N, Yasuda N. Clinics of adhesion [in Japanese]. Tokyo: Ishiyaku Shuppan, 1996.
17. Van Meerbeek B, Inokoshi S, Braem M, et al. Morphological aspects of the resin-dentin interdiffusion zone with different dentin adhesive systems. J Dent Res 1992;71:1530–1540.
18. Gwinnett AJ. Quantitative contribution of resin infiltration/hybridization to denting bonding. Am J Dent 1993;6:7–9.
19. Ingle JI. Endodontics, ed 3. Philadelphia: Lea & Febiger, 1985.
20. Marushima M. Pulpal healing using calcium hydroxide preparation [in Japanese]. J Oral Med 1958;25:149.
21. Yamamura T, Shimono M, Inoue T, et al. How lost dentin is regenerated [in Japanese]. The Quintessence 1986;5(1):14–30.
22. Tsukiboshi M. Color atlas. Treatment planning for traumatized teeth [in Japanese]. Part 1–10. The Quintessence 1994;13(1)–13(10).
23. Tenca JI, Tsamtsouris A. Continued root end development: Apexogenesis and apexification. J Pedod 1978;2:144–157.
24. Gargiulo AW, et al. Dimensions and relations of the dentogingival junction in humans. J Periodontol 1961;32:261.
25. Maynard JG, Wilson RD. Physiologic dimensions of the periodontium significant to the restorative dentist. J Periodontol 1970;50:170.
26. Wilson RD, Maynard JG. Intracrevicular restorative dentistry. Int J Periodontics Restorative Dent 1981;4:34.
27. Nevins M, Mellonig JT. Clinical Approaches and Evidence of Success, vol 1. Periodontal Therapy. Chicago: Quintessence, 1998.
28. Heithersay GS. Combined endodontic-orthodontic treatment of transverse root fractures in the region of the alveolar crest. Oral Surg 1973;36:404–415.
29. Ingber JS. Forced eruption: Part II. A method of treatment for nonrestorable teeth—periodontal and restorative considerations. J Periodontol 1976;47:203–216.
30. Malmgren O, Malmgren B, Frykholm A. Rapid orthodontic extrusion of crown root and cervical root fractured teeth. Endod Dent Traumatol 1991;7:49–54.
31. Kahnberg KE. Surgical extrusion of root-fractured teeth. A follow-up study of two surgical methods. Endod Dent Traumatol 1988;4:85–89.
32. Tegsjö U, Valerius-Olsson H, Olgart K. Intra-alveolar transplantation of teeth with cervical root fractures. Swed Dent J 1978;2:73–82.
33. Ichinokawa H. Micro-structural study of teeth and periodontal tissue change after intentional replantation [in Japanese]. J Operative 1995;38:63–87.
34. Ichinokawa H, Nakagawa K, Isono T, et al. Experimental and pathological study of autotransplantation of teeth. Part I [in Japanese]. J Dent 1996;96:70–71.
35. Friedman N. Periodontal osseous surgery: Osteoplasty and ostectomy. J Periodontol 1955;26:257.
36. Friedman N. Mucogingival surgery. The apically repositioned flap. J Periodontol 1962;33:328–340.
37. Prichard JF. Advanced Periodontal Disease, ed 2. Philadelphia: Saunders, 1972.

38. Frank KL. Therapy for the divergent pulpless tooth by continued apical formation. J Am Dent Assoc 1966;72:87–93.
39. Steiner JC, Van Hassel HJ. Experimental root apexification in primates. Oral Surg 1971;31:409–415.
40. Cved M. Treatment of non-vital permanent incisors with calcium hydroxide. I. Follow-up of periapical repair and apical closure of immature roots. Odontol Revy 1972;23:27.
41. Shinagawa M. Experimental study of apical closure in immature root [in Japanese]. J Kyushu Dent 1980;34:355.
42. Nutting EB, Poe GS. A new combination for bleaching teeth. J South Calif Dent Assoc 1963;31:289–291.
43. Goldstein RE, Garber DA. Complete Dental Bleaching. Chicago: Quintessence, 1995.
44. Andreasen FM, Yu Z, Thomsen BL. The relationship between pulpal dimensions and the development of pulp necrosis after luxation injuries in the permanent dentition. Endod Dent Traumatol 1986;2:90–98.
45. Andreasen FM. Transient apical breakdown and its relation to color and sensibility changes. Endod Dent Traumatol 1986;2: 9–19.
46. Andreasen FM, Yu Z, Thomsen BL, Andreasen PK. The occurrence of pulp canal obliteration after luxation injuries in the permanent dentition. Endod Dent Traumatol 1987;3:103–115.
47. Andreasen FM. Pulpal healing after luxation injuries and root fracture in the permanent dentition. Endod Dent Traumatol 1989;5:111–131.
48. Andreasen JO. The effect of splinting upon periodontal healing after replantation of permanent incisors in monkeys. Acta Odontol Scand 1975;33:313–323.
49. Inoue T, Takahashi K, Maeda T, Shimoji I. Clinical image of transplantation of teeth [in Japanese]. Edited by Tsukiboshi M, et al. The Quintessence 1996 (suppl):36–58.
50. Andreasen JO. Periodontal healing after replantation and autotransplantation of incisors in monkeys. Int J Oral Surg 1981; 10:54–61.
51. Nasjleti CE, Caffesse RG, Castelli WA, Hoke JA. Healing after tooth reimplantation in monkeys. A radioautographic study. Oral Surg 1975;39:361–375.
52. Andreasen JO. A time-related study of periodontal healing and root resorption activity after replantation of mature permanent incisors in monkeys. Swed Dent J 1980;4:101–110.
53. Proye MP, Polson AM. Repair in different zones of the periodontium after tooth reimplantation. J Periodontol 1982;53: 379–389.
54. Araki T, Tsukiboshi M. Science and clinics of autotransplantation of teeth—consideration for regeneration of alveolar bone proper, Sharpey's fiber, blood vessels, and nerve control [in Japanese]. The Quintessence 1992;11(4):725–748.
55. Löe H, Waerhaug J. Experimental replantation of teeth in dogs and monkeys. Arch Oral Biol 1961;3:176–184.
56. Sherman P. Intentional replantation of teeth in dogs and monkeys. J Dent Res 1968;47:1066–1077.
57. Melcher AH. Repair of wounds in the periodontium of the rat. Influence of periodontal ligament on osteogenesis. Arch Oral Biol 1970;15:1183–1204.
58. Andreasen JO, Skougaard MR. Reversibility of surgically induced dental ankylosis in rats. Int J Oral Surg 1972;1:98–102.
59. Andreasen JO. Cementum repair after apicoectomy in humans. Acta Odontol Scand 1973;31:211–221.
60. Line SE, Polson AM, Zander HA. Relationship between periodontal injury, selective cell repopulation and ankylosis. J Periodontol 1974;45:725–730.
61. Andreasen JO. Histometric study of healing of periodontal tissues in rats after a surgical injury, II. Healing events of alveolar bone, periodontal ligaments and cementum. Odontol Rev 1976;27:131–144.
62. Yoshida M. Experimental study of regeneration of cementum, periodontal membrane and alveolar bone in root cavity [in Japanese]. J Dent 1976;76:1179–1222.
63. Andreasen JO, Kristerson L. The effect of limited drying or removal of the periodontal ligament. Periodontal healing after replantation of mature incisors in monkeys. Acta Odontol Scand 1981;39:1–13.
64. Lindskog S, Blomlof L, Hammarström L. Repair of periodontal tissues in vivo and in vitro. J Clin Periodontol 1983;10:188–205.
65. Inoue T, Takei K, Shimono M, Yamamura T, Melcher AH. Regeneration of periodontal ligament in vivo and in vitro. J Dent Res 1987;66:281.
66. Andreasen JO, Borum M, Jacobsen HL, Andreasen FM. Replantation of 400 avulsed permanent incisors. II. Factors related to pulpal healing. Endod Dent Traumatol 1995;11(2):59–68.
67. Andreasen JO, Borum M, Andreasen FM. Replantation of 400 avulsed permanent incisors. III. Factors related to root growth. Endod Dent Traumatol 1995;11(2):69–75.
68. Kristerson L, Andreasen JO. Influence of root development on periodontal and pulpal healing after replantation of incisors in monkeys. Int J Oral Surg 1984;13:313–323.
69. Kristerson L, Andreasen JO. Autotransplantation and replantation of tooth germs in monkeys. Effect of damage to the dental follicle and position of transplant in the alveolus. Int J Oral Surg 1984;13:324–333.
70. Andreasen JO, Kristerson L, Andreasen FM. Damage of the Hertwig's epithelial root sheath: Effect upon root growth after autotransplantation of teeth in monkeys. Endod Dent Traumatol 1988;4:145–151.
71. Andreasen JO, Paulsen HU, Yu Z, et al. A long-term study of 370 autotransplanted premolars. Eur J Orthod 1990;12:3–50.
72. Anderson AW, Sharav Y, Massler M. Reparative dentine formation and pulp morphology. Oral Surg Oral Med Oral Pathol 1968;26:837–847.
73. Skoglund A, Tronstad L, Wallenius K. A microangiographic study of vascular changes in replanted and autotransplanted teeth of young dogs. Oral Surg 1978;45:17–27.
74. Breivik M. Human odontoblast response to tooth replantation. Euro J Orthod 1981;3:95–108.
75. Skoglund A, Hasselgren G, Tronstad L. Oxidoreductase activity in the pulp of replanted and autotransplanted teeth in young dogs. Oral Surg 1981;52:205–209.
76. Monsour FNT, Adkins KF. Aberrations in pulpal histology and dentinogenesis in transplanted erupting teeth. J Oral Maxillofac Surg 1985;43:8–13.
77. Monsour FNT, Adkins KF. Histologic changes following transplantation of developing teeth to more advanced functional positions. Aust Dent J 1987;32:104–109.
78. Kvinnsland I, Heyeraas KJ. Cell renewal and ground substance formation in replanted cat teeth. Acta Odontol Scand 1990;48: 203–215.
79. Gibson ACL. Continued root development after traumatic avulsion of partly-formed permanent incisor. Br Dent J 1969;126: 356–357.

80. Lysell G, Lysell L. A unique case of dilaceration. Odontol Revy 1969;20:43–46.
81. Oliet S. Apexogenesis associated with replantation. A case history. Dent Clin North Am 1974;18:457–464.
82. Barker BCW, Mayne JR. Some unusual cases of apexification subsequent to trauma. Oral Surg Oral Med Oral Pathol 1975;39:144–150.
83. Burley MA, Reece RD. Root formation following traumatic loss of an immature incisor: A case report. Br Dent J 1976;141:315–316.
84. Andreasen JO, Hjörting-Hansen E. Replantation of teeth I. Radiographic and clinical study of 110 human teeth replanted after accidental loss. Acta Odontol Scand 1966;24:263–286.
85. Andreasen JO, Hjörting-Hansen E. Replantation of teeth. II. Histological study of 22 replanted anterior teeth in humans. Acta Odontol Scand 1966;24:287–306.
86. Boyde A, Ali NN, Jones SJ. Resorption of dentine by isolated osteoclasts in vitro. Br Dent J 1984;156:216–220.
87. Andreasen JO. Review of root resorption systems and models. Etiology of root resorption and the homeostatic mechanisms of the periodontal ligament. The Biological Mechanisms of Tooth Eruption and Root Resorption. Birmingham, AL: EBSCO Media, 1988;9–21.
88. Kahn, A, Malone JD. Lineage of bone resorbing cells: Status and prospects of future research. The Biological Mechanisms of Tooth Eruption and Root Resorption. Birmingham, AL: EBSCO Media, 1988;313–319.
89. Andreasen JO. Experimental dental traumatology: Development of a model for external root resorption. Endod Dent Traumatol 1987;3:269–287.
90. Andreasen JO. Relationship between cell damage in the periodontal ligament after replantation and subsequent development of root resorption. Acta Odontol Scand 1981;39:15–25.
91. Andersen L, Johnsson RG, Hammarström L, et al. Evaluation of statistics and desirable experimental design of a histomorphometrical method for studies of root resorption. Endod Dent Traumatol 1987;3:288–295.
92. Jone SJ, Boyde A. The resorption of dentine and cementum in vivo and in vitro. The Biological Mechanisms of Tooth Eruption and Root Resorption. Birmingham, AL: EBSCO Media, 1988; 335–354.
93. Frost HM. Tetracycline-based histological analysis of bone remodeling. Calcif Tissue Res 1969;3:221–237.
94. Iseri H, Solow B. Growth displacement of the maxilla in girls studied by the implant method. Tandloegebladet 1991;94: 839–846.
95. Andreasen JO. The effect of pulp extirpation or root canal treatment on periodontal healing after replantation of permanent incisors in monkeys. J Endod 1981;7:245–252.
96. Andreasen JO. Relationship between surface and inflammatory resorption and changes in the pulp after replantation of permanent incisors in monkeys. J Endod 1981;7:294–301.
97. Andreasen JO. Effect of extra-alveolar period and storage media upon periodontal and pulpal healing after replantation of mature permanent incisors in monkeys. Int Oral Surg 1981;1:43–53.
98. Blomlöf L, Lindskog S, Hammarström L. Periodontal healing of exarticulated teeth stored in milk or saliva. Scand J Dent Res 1981;39:251–259.
99. Blomlöf L, Lindskog S, Andersson L, et al. Storage of experimentally avulsed teeth in milk prior to replantation. J Dent Res 1983;62:912–916.
100. Asai Y, Nakagawa K. Transplantation of teeth. Replantation and preservation of periodontal membrane [in Japanese]. J Japan Dent Soc 1997;50(1):6–16.
101. Asai Y, Nakagawa K, Ichinokawa H, et al. Consideration of preservation solution in transplantation and replantation of teeth [in Japanese]. J Operative 1996;39(suppl):47.
102. Oikarinen VJ, Malmström M. Jaw fractures. A roentgenological and statistical analysis of 1284 cases including a special study of the fracture lines in mandible drawn from orthopantomograms in 660 cases. Suomi Hammaslåäk Toim 1969;65:95–111.
103. Andreasen JO, Sundstrøm B, Ravn JJ. The effect of traumatic injuries to primary teeth on their permanent successors. I. A clinical, radiographic, microradiographic and electron-microscopic study of 117 injured permanent teeth. Scand J Dent Res 1970;79:219–283.
104. Andreasen JO, Ravn JJ. The effect of traumatic injuries to primary teeth on their permanent successors. II. A clinical and radiographic follow-up study of 213 injured teeth. Scand J Dent Res 1970;79:284–294.

Index

References with "t" denote tables; "f" denote figures

D

E

F

G

H

I

L

M

O

P

R

S

T